Covid: A Modern Form of Gu Syndrome

A Chinese Herbal Medicine Theory Handbook

Michael Keane, D.Ac., L.Ac

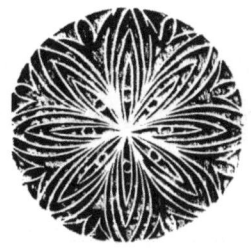

Copyright © 2024 Michael Keane & Michael Keane Creative Studios

All rights reserved. No part of this book may be reproduced in any formor by any means, electronic or mechanical, including photocopying, recording, or by any information storage or retrieval system, without permission.

For any contact or requests please send to:
herbandneedle@protonmail.com

To support my ability to produce future content and publications such as this one, consider donating to me directly via the following sources:

You can find more of my work at the following websites:

www.michaelkeane.art

https://rumble.com/c/MakingArt

www.herbandneedle.org

https://rumble.com/c/HerbAndNeedle

Dedication

To all of the teachers and mentors throughout my journey in the healing arts, thank you.

To all of the people harmed by human hubris and wickedness, may you receive healing.

I would like to thank and acknowledge Dr. Heiner Fruehauf, whose published work on Gu Syndrome inspired and influenced many of the central ideas expressed in this book. His Gu Syndrome formulas and writings have been extremely valuable.

I would also like to acknowledge and express my gratitude to Lorraine Wilcox L.Ac. for sharing many of her wonderful translations of ancient Chinese texts, some of which were utilized in this work.

Warning and Disclaimer

The information in this document is not meant to be used as medical advice. Some of the concepts and ideas are theoretical, hypothetical, and based on tradition. The herbs and herbal formulas discussed in this book are not meant to be considered cures for any disease.

This book is primarily intended as a theory crafting guidebook for experienced practitioners and students of Chinese Herbal Medicine to help in strategizing their treatment plans for long-covid. It is not meant to be considered an end-all be-all text on this topic, but a genuine contribution to the current body of knowledge. The author is not responsible for any unintended consequences arising from the use or misuse of the information contained in this book. It is important to know that there is always the possibility of adverse interactions between herbs and pharmaceutical drugs, and that herbs are potent chemical substances in and of themselves. It is therefore important to always seek professional advice and consultation from qualified herbal medicine practitioners and physicians before using any herbal medicines, including all of the ones discussed in this document.

Contents

9	Introduction
12	Abstract
14	Covid-19
21	Gu Syndrome
28	Covid-19 Gu Syndrome Categories
32	Herbal Treatment Strategies
34	Diaphoretic, Aromatic Herbs to Open the Exterior and Kill Gu Pathogens
39	Herbs to Kill Parasites
48	Herbs to Calm the Spirit and Tonify the Yin
55	Tonify Qi and Blood with Pungent and Detoxifying Substances
63	Invigorate Stagnant Qi and Blood to Expose Lingering Gu Pathogens
73	Su He Tang: A Basis for Modified Gu Formulas
81	Conclusion
83	References

Introduction

What is this book and why did I write it?

This book was written in response to the many people who I come into contact with on a daily basis who have been injured by Covid-19 or Covid-19 vaccines adverse events, and who continue to suffer from debilitating long-Covid symptoms. It is my reaction to this situation in order to help in whatever way I can by transmitting the information and knowledge which I have gathered during my research. It covers and combines the Chinese medicine theory of Gu Syndrome with scientific research which I have compiled on Covid-19 and potential herbal therapies, and presents a new theory for understanding and treating long Covid..

Who am I?

My name is Michael Keane. I am a licensed acupuncturist with doctoral level training in Chinese herbal medicine and acupuncture from the Won Institute of Graduate Studies, where I also teach as an adjunct faculty member. I treat hundreds of patients each month with acupuncture and I have been practicing acupuncture and Chinese herbal medicine for over a decade. I spend a good deal of my free time researching and writing about topics related to acupuncture and medicine, as well as painting and making art. You can find future content and publications at my website, www.herbandneedle.org. My artwork is available on my other website, www.michaelkeane.art.

Who is this book for?

This book is primarily written for practitioners of Chinese herbal medicine and acupuncturists. The goal is to provide theoretical and practical ideas to assist them in treating their patients who are suffering from long-Covid. However, that does not mean that other healthcare professionals or the average person cannot benefit from the information in this book. Anyone with a curious mind might find this book valuable. If you suffer from long-Covid symptoms, you may find a treasure trove of research within this book which might be interesting to you or help you open up new lines of inquiry. I hope it inspires you to seek out and find a licensed acupuncturist with training in Chinese herbal medicine for consultation and treatment. *I always recommend seeking professional consultation in order to avoid potential injury from self-diagnosis and treatment as there are potential dangers associated with the misuse of herbal medicines.*

Abstract

The purpose of this text is to theorize herbal treatment options for long-haul Covid, also known as long-Covid, through the context of a classical Chinese medicine concept known as *Gu Syndrome*. First, we overview the scientific medical literature and illustrate how chronic disease states often can emerge post-virally. Second, we examine the post-viral symptoms of Covid-19 long-Covid syndrome in the current scientific literature. Parallels are drawn between the ancient concept of Gu Syndrome and these chronic Covid long-haul symptoms.

I theorize that the Chinese herbal medicine concept of Gu syndrome may be a useful category for understanding latent viral pathogenicity such as we see in long-Covid. The theory and history of Gu Syndrome is overviewed and important Gu syndrome herbal medicines and formulas are identified and examined. A scientific literature review of each of the individual herbal medicines in Gu formulas is performed in order to assess their relevance in Covid-19 treatment. The intent is to supply practitioners with the ability to apply Gu Syndrome concepts for the development of herbal treatment strategies and custom formulas for their long-haul Covid patients, with a scientific evidence basis whenever possible.

Keywords: *Gu Syndrome, Covid, Covid-19, long-haul Covid, long-Covid, spike protein, Covid vaccine, lingering pathogens, virus, Chinese Herbal Medicine, Su He Tang, Brain Gu, Heart Gu, Lung Gu, Digestive Gu, parasites*

Covid-19

In the wake of the unprecedented Covid-19 pandemic, followed by the wide-scale experimental mRNA vaccination programs utilizing the SARS-CoV-2 spike protein[1], there remains a large population of patients (often called Covid long-haulers) who are experiencing ongoing chronic symptoms colloquially dubbed 'long-Covid'.[2]

It is not uncommon for viral infections to lead to further lingering, chronic diseases after recovery from the acute infection phase. This can be seen for example with Epstein-Barr virus leading to chronic fatigue syndrome.[3] Other pathologies which are thought to arise post-virally include fibromyalgia-like

---

[1] Almehdi, A., Khoder, G., et al. SARS-CoV-2 spike protein: pathogenesis, vaccines, and potential therapies

[2] Bellanti, J.A. The long Covid syndrome: A conundrum for the allergist/immunologist

[3] Bansal, A.S., Bradley, A.A., et al. Chronic fatigue syndrome, the immune system and viral infection

pain, neurological disorders[4], digestive system disorders[5], dermatological disorders, and a variety of autoimmune diseases such as Lupus[6] or Multiple Sclerosis[7]. Viruses can potentially cause the onset of new diseases, accelerate degenerative conditions such as Alzheimer's disease, as well as retrigger issues which have been in remittance, such as various autoimmune disorders.[8] It is also well known that viral agents are implicated in cancer carcinogenesis and actually, viral carcinogenesis is one of the main risk factors for the development of cancer.[9] Beyond the acute phase of a viral infection, a failure or success in treating any latent viral pathogens (and healing the damage done by them) can have life changing long-term consequences on someone's health.

Covid-19 seems to exhibit post-viral persistence reminiscent of a variety of lingering pathologies. "Although the frequency, severity, and potentially the etiology of persistent

---

[4] Wouk, J., Rechenchoski, D.Z., et al. Viral infections and their relationship to neurological disorders

[5] Brown, J.J., et al. A viral trigger for celiac disease

[6] Quaglia, M., Merlotti, G., et al. Viral Infections and Systemic Lupus Erythematosus: New Players in an Old Story

[7] Grigoriadis, N., Hadjigeorgiou, G.M. Virus-mediated autoimmunity in Multiple Sclerosis

[8] Vlieger, L.D., Vandenbroucke, R.E., Hoecke, L.V. Recent insights into viral infections as a trigger and accelerator in alzheimer's disease

[9] Villa, L.L. Viral carcinogenesis: virus implicated in cancer

symptoms can vary, sequelae after Covid-19 appears poised to join the range of other postinfectious syndromes described in the field of infectious diseases."[10] Multiple chronic post-viral Covid-19 pathologies have been identified and given the umbrella title of 'long-haul Covid.' "Clinical symptomatology [of long-Covid] includes fatigue, malaise, dyspnea, defects in memory and concentration and a variety of neuropsychiatric syndromes as the major manifestations, and several organ systems can be involved."[11] It has also been commonplace for patients to experience extended loss of smell and taste, as detailed in a recent Journal of Chinese Medicine case study article.[12] The full range of the underlying pathophysiological mechanisms are poorly understood at the present time and are quite complex. Long-haul Covid-19 is likely to be multifactorial and its manifestations will vary depending upon each individual case and the physiological systems and processes involved.[13]

One hypothesis is that the Covid-19 spike protein, which enables the virus to attach to cells (and which is the basis of the mRNA-based Covid vaccines), is itself a viral pathogen capable of

---

[10] Aucott, J.N., Rebman, A.W. Long-haul Covid: heed the lessons from other infection-triggered illnesses

[11] Mehandru, S., Miriam, M. Pathological sequelae of long-haul Covid

[12] Wang, T. Covid-19-Linked Loss of Smell and Taste: Case Study and Discussion

[13] Maltezou, H.Z., Pavli, A., Tsakris, A. Post-Covid Syndrome: An Insight on Its Pathogenesis

damaging the host and causing pathology. It has been suggested that the spike protein itself may be responsible for the post-acute Covid long-haul syndromes.[14] It is known that the spike protein alone is capable of eliciting cellular signaling events in host cells independent from the rest of the virus.[15][16] Research also suggests that the spike protein is capable of disrupting the blood brain barrier, potentially a neurologically significant finding.[17][18] The spike protein can also cause cardiovascular disease independent of viral infection.[19] If the spike protein is capable of eliciting an acute inflammatory response then it is common sense to consider it to be a toxin. This could explain the overlap seen between common symptoms of Covid-19 and the adverse

---

[14] Theoharides, T. Could SARS-CoV-2 Spike Protein Be Responsible for Long-Covid Syndrome?

[15] Banerjee, S., Wang, X., et al. Comprehensive role of SARS-CoV-2 spike glycoprotein in regulating host signaling pathway

[16] Suzuki, Y.J., Gychna, S.G. SARS-CoV-2 Spike Protein Elicits Cell Signaling in Human Host Cells: Implications for Possible Consequences of Covid-19 Vaccines

[17] DeOre, B.J., Tran, K.A., et al. SARS-CoV-2 Spike Protein Disrupts Blood-Brain Barrier Integrity via RhoA Activation

[18] Erickson, M.A., Rhea, E.M., et al. Interactions of SARS-CoV-2 with the Blood–Brain Barrier

[19] Imig, J.D. SARS-CoV-2 spike protein causes cardiovascular disease independent of viral infection

events which can occur post-vaccination.[20] The common denominator is the SARS-CoV-2 spike protein.[21]

A narrative review article makes a compelling case for this hypothesis, going so far as to coin the term 'Spikeopathy' to describe the spike protein pathogenicity, whether it originates from the virus or is produced by the gene coding of the vaccines. Other authors also echo the same concerns about the dangers of the spike protein, concluding that "evidence strongly supports the possible link between inappropriate expression of S protein in sensitive tissues and subsequent tissue damage."[22]

Spike protein antigen has been found in patients with long-haul post-acute Covid-19 symptoms up to 12 months post-infection, suggesting the possibility of a viral reservoir of Covid-19 spike protein.[23] Circulating spike protein has also been detected in patients who suffer from post-vaccination injuries such as myocarditis.[24] The post-vaccination halflife and concentration of the spike protein in circulation or in organs and

---

[20] Pfizer Responds to Research Claims

[21] Trougakos, I.P., Terpos, E., et al. Adverse effects of Covid-19 mRNA vaccines: the spike hypothesis

[22] Cosentino, M., Marino, F. Understanding the Pharmacology of Covid-19 mRNA Vaccines: Playing Dice with the Spike?

[23] Vanichkachorn, E., Newcomb, R., et al. Persistent circulating SARS-CoV-2 spike is associated with post-acute Covid-19 sequelae

[24] Yonker, L.M., Swank, Z., et al. Circulating Spike Protein Detected in Post-Covid-19 mRNA Vaccine Myocarditis

tissues is not currently known.[25] If the Covid spike protein itself is a viral pathogen capable of pathological damage, then its continued presence in our body is immunologically problematic. It also speaks to the safety signals which have been raised about the experimental vaccines.[26] Recognition of this may be tremendously important towards understanding the etiology of Covid long-haul symptoms and their pathogenesis.[27] Therapeutics (such as herbal medicines) which inhibit the spike protein and aid in its removal from the system would be beneficial and important to identify and to utilize.[28]

I regularly see patients in clinical acupuncture and herbal medicine practice with Covid long-haul symptoms which often manifest as chronic fatigue, 'brain fog' or subjective cognitive impairment, new bodily pains like arthralgias[29] or

---

[25] Trougakos, I.P., Terpos, E., et al. Covid-19 mRNA vaccine-induced adverse effects: unwinding the unknowns

[26] Faksova, K., et al. COVID-19 vaccines and adverse events of special interest: A multinational Global Vaccine Data Network (GVDN) cohort study of 99 million vaccinated individuals

[27] Theoharides, T.C., Conti, P. Be aware of SARS-CoV-2 spike protein: There is more than meets the eye

[28] Suzuki, Y.J. The viral protein fragment theory of Covid-19 pathogenesis

[29] Sapkota, H.R., Nune, A. Long Covid from rheumatology perspective — a narrative review

neuropathies[30], strange new dermatological conditions[31][32] such as hives, the 'classic' altered smell and taste, digestive disturbances[33], neurological disorders[34], headaches and migraines[35], sleep disturbances, tremors or epileptic events, Bell's Palsy, chronic persistent cough, and more. Most patients experience these symptoms post-infection, but many report that their symptoms developed as adverse reactions to vaccination. From a Chinese medicine perspective, I propose that these lingering symptoms (hypothetically caused by latent spike protein pathogen) might be understood as a modern form of Gu Syndrome.

---

[30] Oaklander, A.L., Mills, A.J., et al. Peripheral Neuropathy Evaluations of Patients With Prolonged Long Covid

[31] Panda, M., Dash, S., et al. Dermatological Manifestations Associated with Covid-19 Infection

[32] McMahon, D.E., Gallman, A.E., et al. Long Covid in the skin: a registry analysis of Covid-19 dermatological duration

[33] Bogariu, A.M., Dumitrascu, D.L. Digestive involvement in the Long-Covid syndrome

[34] Stefanou, M., Palaiodimou, L., et al. Neurological manifestations of long-Covid syndrome: a narrative review

[35] Chhabra, N., Grill, M.F., Singh, R.B.H. Post-Covid Headache: A Literature Review

Gu Syndrome

The Chinese character for Gu is depicted by a bowl of worms, snakes, or venomous creatures, giving a visual of a thriving population of malevolent, miasmic influences (possibly parasites, worms, poisonous snakes, insects like centipedes or scorpions, fungi and mold, etc.) thought to be the hidden cause of strange pathologies.

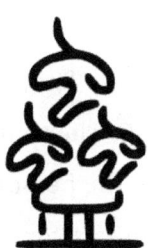

Traditional Chinese seal script character for 'Gu'[36]

---

[36] Gu (poison). Wikipedia

Historically, Gu was sometimes thought of as a 'possession syndrome', a kind of black magic.[37] Ancient texts tell us that Gu syndromes were commonly human-made and sometimes purposefully used to poison people via food or drink.

Zhubing Yuanhou Lun edited by Chao Yuanfang (610 CE, Sui) Volume 24, Section 13: Gu Infixation Symptoms:

"Infixation means residing. It refers to a disease that is continuously stagnant and stays to reside within the patient. It is easy for a person with infixation to be near death. Gu is in the category of gathered snakes and *chong* [creepy crawly parasites/insects]. They are contained in a bowl and made to feed on each other. The one that remains alive in the end is the Gu, and it can mutate. People who make it treat it with respectful attention. They use the toxins to harm others. Many employ it by putting it in food and drink. People struck by Gu have heart oppression or abdominal pain. They die when it completely eats away the five Zang [organs]. There are chronic and acute types. The acute type acts quickly; the person dies within ten to twenty days. The chronic type can last for years, traveling around the abdomen. Often, physical strength is exhausted, and the bones and joints feel heavy. During episodes, there is vexation of the

---

[37] Fruehauf, Heiner. Driving Out Demons and Snakes: A Forgotten Clinical Approach to Chronic Parasitism

heart region and abdominal pain. Everything the person eats also mutates into Gu, gradually invading and completely consuming the organs until the victim dies. Once dead, the disease flows and infixes into nearby people, polluting them, so it is called Gu Infixation."[38]

> *Jingyue Quanshu by Zhang Jeibin (1624, Ming)*
> *Volume 35: Excerpts on Gu Toxins:*
>
> "Gu is a kind of toxin. It rarely appears in the central plains of China. It is transmitted from generation to generation in Guangxi and Guangdong by people in the remote mountains. On the fifth day of the lunar month, they fill a vessel with three things together: venomous snakes, centipedes, and toads. They allow them to devour each other and wait until only one is left alive. This one is used as the Gu. It is also called *taosheng*. They secretly put Gu in the food and drink of someone they want to harm. The person is struck by the toxins. They will have illness and pain in their heart region and abdomen as if the Gu were gnawing on them. They have both vomiting and diarrhea that looks like decayed silk floss. If it is not treated right away, it eats the five Zang of the victim and they die. Some die ten to twenty days later. Beyond this, there is a chronic type that can take

---

[38] Translation by Lorraine Wilcox, Gu Toxins. Youtube.

years. Qi and blood become exhausted. They die after it has completely eaten their five Zang."

"It is said that in Lingnang (Guangxi and Guangdong) people kill venomous snakes and cover them with herbs. They sprinkle water on it. After a few days, fungus grows. They powder the fungus and mix it with rice wine to poison people. There is no suffering in the beginning, but when they drink wine again later, the poison works and they die."[39]

These descriptions of Gu syndrome evoke ideas of a sort of pre-modern biological terrorism, the use of pestilential forces, poisonous toxins, and man-made pathogens to engender disease. Given the obscure origins of Covid-19 and the unresolved theories about gain-of-function research and the potential of a lab leak origin, these correlations are certainly intriguing at the very least.[40]

Though these descriptions focus on the pathogens entering the body via intentional poisoning of food and drink, Gu pathogens can certainly enter the body through other means. The above passages allude to contagious properties, noting that it can pass between people. Once it has infiltrated a host, whether there is a deadly acute phase or not, Gu becomes

---

[39] Ibid.
[40] Maxmen, A., Mallapaty, S. The Covid lab-leak hypothesis: what scientists do and don't know

infixated. I take the meaning of this to be that the pathogens become deeply entrenched and difficult to fully remove. Importantly, the texts tell us that some Gu are chronic syndromes, with slow, mysterious, degenerative effects over time.

More recently, Dr. Heiner Fruehauf utilizes Gu syndrome as a concept to understand a variety of poorly understood and hard to treat modern degenerative diseases. He says, "Gu syndrome actually means that your system is hollowed out from the inside out by dark yin forces that you cannot see."[41] For example, he applies this concept to cases such as Lyme disease, AIDS, herpes, Coxsackievirus, systemic yeast infections, parasites, amoebic disorders, and the strange autoimmune, inflammatory, neurological, fatigue-like symptoms which many people develop as chronic conditions. Since Gu syndrome is a hidden pathogenic force causing degenerative changes and strange illnesses of unknown or unclear origins, he believes it should be considered in these types of patients.

To quote a Journal of Chinese Medicine article on Gu Syndrome called, 'Driving Out Demons and Snakes: A Forgotten Clinical Approach to Chronic Parasitism by Dr. Heiner Fruehauf: "Master Ranxi (Ranxi Daoren), a Qing Dynasty Daoist healer who

---

[41] Fruehauf, Heiner. Gu Syndrome: An In-depth Interview with Heiner Fruehauf

specialised in the treatment of Gu syndrome, pointed out that chronic parasite infections are very resilient and hard to resolve thoroughly. "Gu toxins that have entered the core of a person's being can be compared to oil seeping into flour - it is everywhere and cannot be separated out". He notes that although this disorder is serious and affects the patient on all levels of existence, he or she may well live with this situation forever without necessarily dying from it. He compares the situation to a tree that hosts birds and insects in various parts of its structure."[42]

I believe this same line of thinking can be applied to long-haul Covid-19, as it displays all the signs of a lingering, chronic Gu pathogen. Let us consider the Covid spike protein which, whether contracted externally or delivered internally by a vaccine, has the energetic quality of being a spike. This means that its nature is one of stickiness, sharpness, pokiness, and it is thus with some level of difficulty that it is cleared and removed from the body. As a metaphor, one might consider the spikes of burrs which stick to our clothes after a hike through the woods. They take a level of persistence to remove them from our garments. In the same vein, the body may have trouble removing the spike proteins which become embedded within the cellular

---

[42] Fruehauf, Heiner. Driving Out Demons and Snakes: A Forgotten Clinical Approach to Chronic Parasitism

spaces of the body's tissues. Even when the acute phase is over and we think that the pathogen may be gone, some may yet remain within the crevices and dark hidden spaces.

We have seen that the spike protein continues circulating in our system for an unknown period of time, both post-Covid infection and post-vaccination. Any lingering spikes might cause chronic issues due to inflammatory immune and autoimmune responses (heat), congestion or coagulation of the cellular spaces (blood stagnation or phlegm), and other malign processes typical of chronic illnesses that arise when a pathogen lies hidden but ever present in our body. It also leaves the organism vulnerable to other opportunistic pathogens due to a weakened and preoccupied immune function. From a Chinese medicine perspective, it is likely that there will be symptoms of inflammatory heat, elements of residual blood stagnation and phlegm which form, as well as deep underlying deficiency. These processes are all downstream of the continued presence of the lingering pathogen.

Covid-19 Gu Syndrome Categories

The following theoretical categories should not be considered static or exclusive from each other. Gu syndrome may have chronic systemic effects which overlap in their shared symptomatology. However, we might consider seemingly distinct types centered on certain physiological systems and constellations of symptoms. Dr. Heiner Fruehauf differentiates between two primary types of Gu syndrome which he observes called Brain Gu and Digestive Gu.[43] These systems are also implicated in many long-Covid clinical cases which I see. In light of the unique ways in which Covid-19 enters, attacks, and

---

[43] Fruehauf, Heiner. Gu Syndrome: An In-depth Interview with Heiner Fruehauf

damages the body, I propose that we also consider two other potential affected systems: Lung Gu[44] and Heart Gu[45].

1. Lung / Respiratory Gu
(consider in respiratory infection cases)
2. Heart / Cardiovascular Gu
(consider in post-vaccination cases)
3. Brain / Neurological Gu
(often part of the constellation of symptoms)
4. Digestive Gu
(often part of the constellation of symptoms)

Common sense says that the pathway in which the pathogen enters the body and where it lingers and causes damage determines the systems primarily affected. We might consider the infectious respiratory route primarily as Lung Gu if a patient manifests with continued respiratory pathologies. Heart (or cardiovascular) Gu might arise post-vaccination due to the systemic distribution of spike protein throughout the body via the cardiovascular system. Symptoms of both Brain and Digestive Gu Syndrome will likely manifest prominently as part of a patient's overall constellation of symptoms as well. Chronic

---

[44] Sanchez-Ramirez, D.C., Normand, K., et al. Long-Term Impact of Covid-19: A Systematic Review of the Literature and Meta-Analysis

[45] Tobler, D.L., Pruzansky, A.J., et al. Long-Term Cardiovascular Effects of Covid-19: Emerging Data Relevant to the Cardiovascular Clinician

fatigue and brain fog are two of the most common complaints I see. These symptom constellations are not mutually exclusive, but often overlap and manifest in tandem with each other to varying degrees. In some cases, Gu Syndrome could be systemic throughout all systems, and some patients may present with symptoms which fall into each system or category. The following Venn diagrams are examples of potential constellations of symptoms from long-haul Covid Gu syndromes:

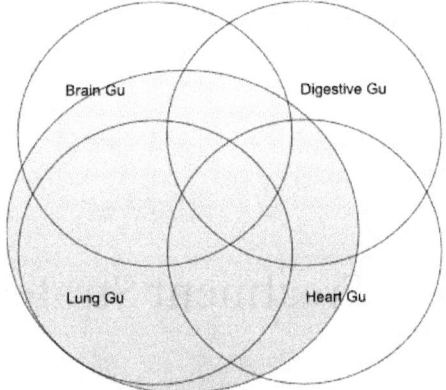

Lung Gu symptom constellation
post-respiratory Covid infection

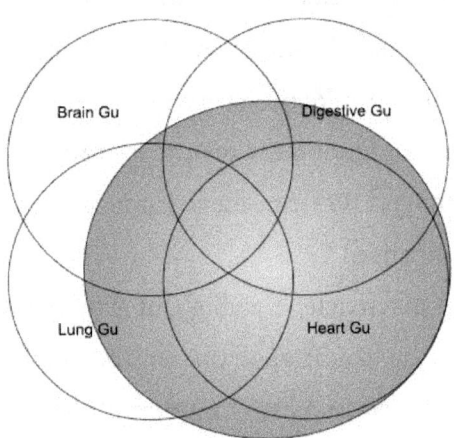

Heart Gu symptom constellation
post-Covid vaccination reaction

31

Herbal Treatment Strategies

In this section we consider a number of classical Chinese herbs and treatment categories which have been used for Gu Syndromes in the past and the present, with a special intention of driving out chronic hidden retainment of the Covid spike protein. Any relevant scientific research relating these herbs to Covid will be included. As noted by Dr. Heiner Fruehauf, one of the main concepts to keep in mind with Gu herbs is that "constant herbal fumigation makes the system uninhabitable for any kind of pathogen. We can look at most of these herbs as a sort of internal incense."[46]

To quote his article, 'Driving Out Demons and Snakes' on Gu Syndrome: "The traditional Gu approach, therefore, is the result of a carefully crafted program that utilises i. blood movers

---

[46] Fruehauf, Heiner. Gu Syndrome: An In-depth Interview with Heiner Fruehauf

to "push through barriers of accumulated phlegm and blood, exposing the parasites and making them vulnerable for attack"; ii. aromatic antiparasitic herbs that create an uninviting milieu for the invaders; and finally iii. tonic substances that stimulate the body's own scavengers which feed on foreign organisms. For each category, moreover, Gu therapists chose to employ herbs that were also known to be anti-parasitic in one way or another."[47]

Some of these herbs may have properties and actions from multiple categories, so their categorical placement should be taken with a grain of salt. Many can be flexibly combined, added, or removed depending on the constellation of symptoms in each case. Ideally, this list is meant to guide practitioners in the creation of custom herbal formulas for their individual Covid / Gu cases, not as static formulas to be applied to every case.

---

[47] Ibid.

Diaphoretic, Aromatic Herbs To Open the Exterior and Kill Gu Pathogens

The most important herbal category for Gu syndrome is that of diaphoretic, aromatic herbs. "Perilla (both leaf and seed - Zi Su Ye and Su Zi), Bo He and Bai Zhi particularly are extremely visible in traditional Gu formulas. Their sweat-inducing properties are much weaker than other diaphoretics like Ma Huang (Herba Ephedrae) or Gui Zhi (Ramulus Cinnamomi Cassiae), and they are imbued with a strong aromatic fragrance - a penetrating yang energy that, like a diffusive light, is able to permeate the darkest crevasses of the body where the Gu pathogens hide out. For the same reason, acupressure with mint oil was often recommended. Traditional Gu specialists honoured this saturating effect by creating a new medicinal category for this group of herbs, namely "open the exterior with snake killing herbs" (shashe fabiao)."[48]

Zi Su Ye (Perilla Leaf)

Zi Su Ye has an aromatic nature and can 'revivify' the entire body, implied by the character 'Su' of its name.[49] Interestingly, a 2021 study found that Perilla leaf extract successfully inhibits Covid viral entry, perhaps due to an effect on the spike protein. It reduced viral replication and decreased cytokine and inflammatory reactions to the virus.[50]

Bai Zhi (Angelica Dahuricae Radix)

Bai Zhi is helpful for opening the orifices, especially the nasal passages[51], which is worth noting for patients with smell and taste deficiency. It has known anti-viral properties[52], and is

---

[48] Ibid.

[49] Bensky, et al. Materia Medica

[50] Tang, W., Tsai, H., et al. Perilla (Perilla frutescens) leaf extract inhibits SARS-CoV-2 via direct virus inactivation

[51] Bensky, et al. Materia Medica

[52] Lee, B.W., Ha, T.K.Q., et al. Antiviral activity of furanocoumarins isolated from Angelica dahurica against influenza a viruses H1N1 and H9N2

rich in coumarins, volatile oils, and other phytochemicals with potential usage against Covid.[53][54]

Bo He (Menthae Haplocalysis Herba)

Bo He is a useful aromatic herb whose "lightness floats and ascends while its sweet aroma unblocks the orifices."[55] The Materia Medica describes it as having the ability to 'expel turbid filth' as well as having the ability to treat sores and rashes. Consider it even more in patients with post-Covid skin or digestive issues.[56]

Tulsi (Ocimum Sanctum)

Tulsi, also known as Holy Basil, is an aromatic Ayurvedic herb from the Mint family which is renowned for its adaptogenic, immunomodulatory, cardioprotective, antiviral, and diaphoretic properties.[57] It is hailed as an 'elixir of life' in Ayurvedic

---

[53] Zhao, H., Feng, Y., et al. Bai Zhi (Angelica Dahuricae Radix)

[54] Abrahim, M.A.A., Mohamed, E.A.R., et al. Rutin and flavone analogs as prospective SARS-CoV-2 main protease inhibitors: In silico drug discovery study

[55] Bensky, et al. Materia Medica

[56] Ibid.

[57] Shree, P., Mishra, P., et al. Targeting Covid-19 (SARS-CoV-2) main protease through active phytochemicals of ayurvedic medicinal plants – Withania somnifera (Ashwagandha), Tinospora cordifolia (Giloy) and Ocimum sanctum (Tulsi) – a molecular

medicine.[58] Although it is not a traditional Gu herb, I chose to include it due to its broad adaptogenic properties. It is often used for its cardiovascular benefits, anxiolytic and antidepressant properties, and its benefits for memory and cognition.[59] It has powerful phytochemicals with anti-Covid actions such as Eugenol[60] and Ursolic Acid.[61]

Gao Ben (Rhizoma et Radix Ligustici Sinensis) & Sheng Ma (Rhizoma Cimicifugae)

Along with Bai Zhi, we might consider the use of Gao Ben and Sheng Ma. These herbs have an ascending nature and are often used to treat headaches.[62] Long Covid patients commonly present with headaches, whether of new onset or of a resurgent

---

       docking study

[58] Ibid.

[59] Cohen, M.M. Tulsi - Ocimum sanctum: A herb for all reasons

[60] Paidi, R.K., Jana, M., et al. Eugenol, a Component of Holy Basil (Tulsi) and Common Spice Clove, Inhibits the Interaction Between SARS-CoV-2 Spike S1 and ACE2 to Induce Therapeutic Responses

[61] Al-Kuraishy, H.M., Al-Gareeb, A.I., et al. The possible role of ursolic acid in Covid-19: A real game changer

[62] Bensky, et al. Materia Medica

nature post-Covid, so these herbs might be applicable in those cases.[63]

Gao Ben directs Qi upwards to the vertex, treating Taiyang and Du Mai headaches. Sheng Ma and Bai Zhi can treat Yangming frontal headaches.[64] Chuan Xiong is able to treat Shaoyang temporal headaches and can also be added.[65] Accurate differential diagnoses can help us pick which of these herbs is most beneficial for each individual case.

Lian Qiao (Forsythia Fructus)

Lian Qiao is another useful herb in this category, especially when heat is an issue. For example, wind-heat headaches or inflammatory body conditions, rashes and dermatological flare ups, could be signs that this herb should be included in a Gu formula. Lian Qiao can also be useful for draining heat from the Heart, which might manifest as manic or disturbed post-Covid mental emotional signs or symptoms.[66]

---

[63] Chhabra, N., Grill, M.F., Singh, R.B.H. Post-Covid Headache: A Literature Review
[64] Bensky, et al. Materia Medica
[65] Ibid.
[66] Ibid.

Herbs to Kill Parasites

A feature of Gu Syndrome is the tendency for synergistic cooperation between parasitic Gu pathogens to generate a symbiotic relationship whereby "multiple types of infections that all thrive upon each other's existence symbiotically assist each other in the process of feeding upon their more and more deficient host."[67] Therefore, herbs with antiparasitic properties are employed. These herbs are known to help clear out these parasitic pathogens.

---

[67] Fruehauf, H.. An Ancient Solution for Modern Diseases: "Gu Syndrome" and Chronic Inflammatory Diseases with Autoimmune Complications (An Interview with Heiner Fruehauf)

Raw Garlic (Da Suan)

Garlic is a preeminent herb for dispelling parasites. As a functional food, it is rich in compounds with anti-Covid potential.[68] "Raw garlic (Da Suan), in particular the single-clove purple garlic from Sichuan, is often recommended as the most effective single remedy for Gu syndrome."[69]

Garlic has been studied and found to modulate proinflammatory cytokines and many immunological abnormalities characteristic of Covid-19 and it has been recommended as a prophylactic, as its general antiviral properties have been demonstrated.[70] It has the ability to decrease the proinflammatory adipose enzyme leptin, which may contribute to more severe Covid-19 disease and comorbidity in obese patients.[71]

---

[68] Khubber, S., Hashemifesharaki, R., et al. Garlic (Allium sativum L.): a potential unique therapeutic food rich in organosulfur and flavonoid compounds to fight with Covid-19

[69] Fruehauf, Heiner. Driving Out Demons and Snakes: A Forgotten Clinical Approach to Chronic Parasitism

[70] Donma, M.M., Donma, O. The effects of allium sativum on immunity within the scope of Covid-19 infection

[71] Maurya, R., Sebastian, P., et al. Covid-19 Severity in Obesity: Leptin and Inflammatory Cytokine Interplay in the Link Between High Morbidity and Mortality

Yu Jin (Tuber Curcumae)

Yu Jin should be considered due to its ability to break up blood stasis, move the Qi and blood, and cool the blood.[72] I would consider it in most cases involving pain, such as headaches, arthralgias, myalgias, etc. If it is suspected that there is sustained damage from the virus, it may help to cool the inflammatory heat and move the stagnant Qi and blood. One of the primary active constituents of Yu Jin is Curcumin. Curcumin has been shown to have important immunological effects, making it a potentially useful prophylactic for Covid-19.[73] It has antiviral, anti-inflammatory, anticoagulatory, antiplatelet, and cytoprotective properties.[74] Since it can clear heat from the Heart and helps move stagnant Liver Qi, I would also consider it in patients exhibiting various mental emotional issues such as anxiety, agitation, or neuropsychiatric symptoms.[75]

---

[72] Bensky, et al. Materia Medica

[73] Thimmulappa, R.K., Mudnakudu-Nagaraju, K.K., et al. Antiviral and immunomodulatory activity of curcumin: A case for prophylactic therapy for Covid-19

[74] Rattis, B.A.C., Ramos, S.G., Celes, M.R. Curcumin as a Potential Treatment for Covid-19

[75] Bensky, et al. Materia Medica

Jin Yin Hua (Japonica Flos)

Jin Yin Hua is useful in cases where there is heat or chronic inflammation in the Lungs and Stomach. It is well known for its cool nature and its ability to clear heat and toxins. But it is also sweet and is able to tonify deficiency. I think this makes it a particularly well suited herb for weakened long-haul Covid-19 patients. Research shows that Jin Yin Hua exerts numerous anti-inflammatory, anti-viral, and immunoregulatory actions through various pathways, as well as exerts neuroprotective, cardioprotective, hepatoprotective, and antipyretic effects. The phytochemicals of Jin Yin Hua have been shown to be active on multiple levels against Covid-19.[76] Jin Yin Hua has also been shown to interrupt the spike protein binding to cellular Ace2 receptors, the primary binding point for spike protein.[77] The main flavonoid in Jin Yin Hua, Luteolin, has been recommended as an alternative for long-Covid brain fog.[78]

Jin Yin Hua combined with Huang Qi, another Gu herb from the tonifying category, have been shown *in vitro* to reduce

---

[76] Zhao, H., Zeng, S., et al. Updated pharmacological effects of Lonicerae japonicae flos, with a focus on its potential efficacy on coronavirus disease-2019 (Covid-19)

[77] Zhao, H., Zeng, S., et al. Lonicerae Japonicae Flos Attenuates Neutrophilic Inflammation by Inhibiting Oxidative Stress

[78] Theoharides, T., Cholevas, C., et al. Long-Covid syndrome-associated brain fog and chemofog: Luteolin to the rescue

inflammatory cytokines as well as inhibit the spike protein.[79] Jin Yin Hua is also commonly combined with Lian Qiao, an herb from the exterior-opening snake-killing category just mentioned above. Together, they are also the two chief herbs found in Yin Qiao San (Honeysuckle and Forsythia Powder), forming a potent Dui Yao combination.[80] Yin Qiao San itself has been explored as a potential Covid treatment.[81] Together, they can be useful for symptoms involving heat, inflammation, and toxicity.

Ding Xiang / Clove (Caryophylli Flos)

Due to its acrid hot nature and its ability to dispel cold dampness, I would consider Ding Xiang for a patient displaying signs of cold or damp cold, especially in the Spleen and Stomach, such as with nausea and vomiting, epigastric pains, or diarrhea. In the contexts of Covid, research into clove has focused on its anti-viral, anti-inflammatory, and antithrombotic effects.[82] Multiple phytochemicals in cloves have been investigated as

---

[79] Yeh, Y., Doan, L.H., et al. Honeysuckle (Lonicera japonica) and Huangqi (Astragalus membranaceus) Suppress SARS-CoV-2 Entry and Covid-19 Related Cytokine Storm in Vitro

[80] Bensky, et al. Materia Medica

[81] Lin, H., Wang, X., et al. Exploring the treatment of Covid-19 with Yinqiao powder based on network pharmacology

[82] Vicidomini, C., Roviello, V., Roviello, G.N. Molecular Basis of the Therapeutical Potential of Clove (Syzygium aromaticum L.) and Clues to Its Anti-Covid-19 Utility

potentially useful against Covid. Eugenol has been observed to inhibit the Covid spike protein.[83] Myricetin reduced viral replication and reduced pulmonary inflammation.[84] The flavonoid kaempferol has been specifically discussed in conjunction with ophthalmological and retinal diseases associated with post-Covid, such as macular degeneration.[85]

Qing Hao (Artemisiae Annuae Herba)

Qing Hao is very useful for clearing yin deficiency heat without injuring the Qi, Blood, or Yin, making it a somewhat gentle herb which can be used in deficiency cases.[86] It is appropriate when a patient's symptoms relate to injured Yin, which can manifest as chronic inflammation which gets worse in the evening. Since it cools the Blood and vents heat and pathogens from the Yin level, it can be useful for dermatological conditions.[87]

---

[83] Paidi, R.K., Jana, M., et al. Eugenol, a Component of Holy Basil (Tulsi) and Common Spice Clove, Inhibits the Interaction Between SARS-CoV-2 Spike S1 and ACE2 to Induce Therapeutic Responses

[84] Xiao, T., Cui, M., et al. Myricetin Inhibits SARS-CoV-2 Viral Replication by Targeting Mpro and Ameliorates Pulmonary Inflammation

[85] Firaz, A., et al. Covid-19 and retinal degenerative diseases: Promising link "Kaempferol"

[86] Bensky, et al. Materia Medica

[87] Ibid.

Qing Hao has also been extensively studied with regards to its anti-viral, anti-malarial, and anti-Covid properties. It has many phytochemicals which have been shown to potentially inhibit Covid through multiple pathways, including inhibiting the attachment of spike proteins.[88] A principle phytochemical, the sesquiterpene Artemisenin and its derivatives, have been suggested as potential treatments for Covid.[89] They showed promising actions for inhibition of the spike protein binding domains.[90]

He Zi (Fructus Terminaliae Chebulae)

He Zi is an herb which can be used to transform phlegm and stop coughing and wheezing. It directs the Lung Qi downwards and clears phlegm and fire from the Lungs.[91] It is an antiparasitic herb to consider for a patient who has chronic post-

---

[88] Fuzimoto, A.D. An overview of the anti-SARS-CoV-2 properties of Artemisia annua, its antiviral action, protein-associated mechanisms, and repurposing for Covid-19 treatment

[89] Agrawal, P.K., Agrawal, C., Blunden, G. Artemisia Extracts and Artemisinin-Based Antimalarials for Covid-19 Management: Could These Be Effective Antivirals for Covid-19 Treatment?

[90] Sehaila, M., Chemat, S. Antimalarial-agent artemisinin and derivatives portray more potent binding to Lys353 and Lys31-binding hotspots of SARS-CoV-2 spike protein than hydroxychloroquine: potential repurposing of artenimol for Covid-19

[91] Bensky, et al. Materia Medica

Covid Lung Gu where phlegm needs to be expelled. It is astringent and it binds the intestines, so it may be useful for patients with chronic diarrhea, but there may be better herbs to choose for patients with chronic constipation.

Shi Chang Pu (Acori Tatarinowii Rhizoma)

Shi Chang Pu is usually in the category of herbs which aromatically open the orifices, making it another powerful aromatic fumigant. It is said to dislodge phlegm and remove 'filth' and turbid dampness, especially from the middle burner. It is useful for clearing phlegm that is misting the Heart and it opens the senses and clears the mind.[92] It will aid in opening and clearing phlegm which is harboring lingering Gu pathogens. I think this is a top herb for patients with Brain Gu and symptoms of brain fog, sensory disturbances, and mental emotional disturbances. It can awaken the Spleen Qi and benefits the middle burner, so it can be useful for Digestive Gu as well.[93] It also promotes blood flow.[94] It has many bioactive phytochemicals and has been studied for its neuroprotective

---

[92] Ibid.
[93] Fruehauf, Heiner. Gu Syndrome: An In-depth Interview with Heiner Fruehauf
[94] Bensky, et al. Materia Medica

properties[95] and its multipathway prevention and treatment of stroke.[96]

Ku Shen (Sophorae Flavescentis Radix)

Ku Shen is an antiparasitic herb with bitter, cold, cooling properties. It is very useful for treating damp heat conditions which manifest in the urinary system, digestive tract, or Liver.[97] There have been cases where patients have developed digestive disorders such as ulcerative colitis post-Covid.[98] I would consider Ku Shen as a Digestive Gu herb for patients with definite signs of damp heat and toxin in their digestive tract, urinary tract, etc.

---

[95] Lam, K.Y.C., Chen, J., et al. Asarone from Acori Tatarinowii Rhizoma Potentiates the Nerve Growth Factor-Induced Neuronal Differentiation in Cultured PC12 Cells: A Signaling Mediated by Protein Kinase A

[96] Liu, F., Zhao, Q., et al. Revealing the Pharmacological Mechanism of Acorus tatarinowii in the Treatment of Ischemic Stroke Based on Network Pharmacology

[97] Bensky, et al. Materia Medica

[98] Kartsoli, S., Vrakas, S., et al. Ulcerative colitis after SARS-CoV-2 infection

Herbs to Calm the Spirit and Tonify the Yin

Many of these herbs are useful for tonifying the Yin of a patient, which can often manifest as jitteriness, nervousness, and nervous system issues. On this topic, Dr. Heiner Fruehauf says, "I look at yin tonics, particularly the yin of the Lung, as a kind of protective sheathing around the nerves. When people say their nerves are fried, it is really the yin of the Lung that has been compromised."[99]

Bai He (Bulbus Lilii)

Bai He is an important herb to consider in post-Covid patients with Lung Gu. In terms of Yin deficiency, particularly Lung Yin deficiency, Bai He is a preeminent herb. Since Covid is

---

[99] Fruehauf, Heiner. Gu Syndrome: An In-depth Interview with Heiner Fruehauf

particularly damaging to the Lungs and respiratory system, Bai He can be a useful medicinal to help restore a depleted Lung Yin. In the Shang Han Lun, Bai He was also used to treat 'Lily Disease', a sort of mental emotional imbalance caused by Lung Yin deficiency.[100]

Sha Shen (Radix Glehniae Littoralis)

Sha Shen is another herb which is useful for tonifying the Lung Yin and generating fluids.[101] I would add this herb in a formula for symptoms of dryness such as a dry cough with little phlegm, constipation, dry skin, a tendency towards thirst, or other signs and symptoms that the fluids have been injured. It also has strong immunoregulatory, anti-inflammatory, and neuroprotective attributes.[102]

Huang Jing (Rhizome Polygonati)

Dr. Heiner Fruehauf describes Huang Jing as a "Daoist herb often used by hermits in the countryside in southern and southwest China to ward off parasites and to calm the nervous

---

[100] Ibid.
[101] Bensky, et al. Materia Medica
[102] Yang, M., Xue, L., et al. Ethnopharmacology, Phytochemistry, and Pharmacology of the Genus Glehnia: A Systematic Review

system."[103] Huang Jing nourishes the Yin, Qi, and Jing, and is useful for Lung Yin deficiency, particularly when there is a dry cough - a symptom commonly seen in Covid long-haul patients. It is also useful for the Spleen and Stomach Qi, and should be considered when a patient is fatigued, has a loss of taste or appetite, or is more on the loose stool side of the spectrum.[104] When combined with Bai He and Sha Shen, it can be guided to the Lungs.

Huang Jing has been considered to have promising antiviral effects against Covid-19, particularly due to its phytochemical Diosgenin.[105] Diosgenin is being studied for its potential uses for degenerative neurological diseases like Alzheimer's disease[106], which is a serious concern due to Covid-19's ability to accelerate the progression of this disease in vulnerable patients.[107]

---

[103] Bensky, et al. Materia Medica
[104] Ibid.
[105] Mu, C., Sheng, Y., et al. Potential compound from herbal food of Rhizoma Polygonati for treatment of Covid-19 analyzed by network pharmacology: Viral and cancer signaling mechanisms
[106] Cai, B., Zhang, Y., et al. Therapeutic Potential of Diosgenin and Its Major Derivatives against Neurological Diseases: Recent Advances
[107] Naughton, S.X., Raval, U., Pasinetti, G.M. Potential Novel Role of Covid-19 in Alzheimer's Disease and Preventative Mitigation Strategies

Xuan Shen (Radix Scrophularia ningpoensis)

Xuan Shen clears heat and cools the Blood as well as nourishes the Yin and Fluids. It enters the Lungs and can be used to clear heat and moisten the Lung Yin, perhaps combined with Bai He. Xuan Shen is also commonly combined with Sheng Di Huang to nourish the Yin and clear heat from the Blood, they are a good combination for patients with Yin deficiency heat symptoms. Xuan Shen can be used in cases with dermatological manifestations.[108] It has detoxifying, mass-reducing qualities.[109] It has been shown to exhibit anti-inflammatory, immune enhancing, cardioprotective, neuroprotective, and cognitive enhancing effects, making it a useful and flexible herb for a variety of post-Covid manifestations.[110] It is rich in many biologically active phytochemicals.[111]

---

[108] Bensky, et al. Materia Medica

[109] Zhang, Q., Liu, A., Wang, Y. Scrophularia ningpoensis Hemsl: a review of its phytochemistry, pharmacology, quality control and pharmacokinetics

[110] Lee, H., Kim, H., et al. Scrophulariae Radix: An Overview of Its Biological Activities and Nutraceutical and Pharmaceutical Applications

[111] Ren, D., Shen, Z., et al. Pharmacology, phytochemistry, and traditional uses of Scrophularia ningpoensis Hemsl

Sheng Di Huang (Radix Rehmanniae Glutinosae)

Sheng Di Huang cools heat and the blood and the nutritive levels of the body. It nourishes the Yin and Fluids and moistens dryness. It can be very useful to clear heat which arises from Yin deficiency, which might manifest as insomnia, night sweats, dry mouth, continuous low grade fever or returning inflammation. Combine it with Qing Hao for smoldering heat which returns at night.[112] It is often combined with Xuan Shen to nourish the Yin, Blood, and Fluids.

Sheng Di Huang can also be combined with Bai He to create the Shang Han Lun formula Bai He Di Huang Tang, which is classically used for a variety of mental emotional disorders, cognitive issues, and sensorimotor dysfunctions. Bai He Di Huang Tang is used when pathogenic heat enters the Heart and Lungs and the Blood and creates mental emotional and psychic disorder, often in the wake of an externally contracted disease.[113] This combination has a multicomponent effect on depression.[114]

---

[112] Bensky, et al. Materia Medica

[113] Scheid, V., et al. Formulas and Strategies

[114] Zhong, H., Xue, X., et al. Integrated analysis of the chemical-material basis and molecular mechanisms for the classic herbal formula of Lily Bulb and Rehmannia Decoction in alleviating depression

This sort of patient might have a slightly rapid pulse, dark urine, a bitter taste in the mouth, and a tongue with little coating.

Xi Yang Shen (Panacis Quinquefolii)

Xi Yang Shen is also known as American Ginseng. It has a cooler nature than Ren Shen, and it tonifies the Yin and the Fluids as well as the Qi, entering the Heart, Kidneys, and Lungs.[115] Xi Yang Shen is a useful addition when Covid-19 has done damage to the Lung Yin and the fluids, or if there are symptoms of Yin deficiency heat. Add it in cases with lingering cough and chronic fatigue.

Covid can cause damage to the Heart and circulatory system, and the Ginsenosides found in Xi Yang Shen have been considered for their cardioprotective properties.[116] It has anti inflammatory, immune enhancing, anticancer, and antiviral properties.[117] It is considered to be an herb which has beneficial

---

[115] Bensky, et al. Materia Medica

[116] Hossain, M.A., Kim, J. Possibility as role of ginseng and ginsenosides on inhibiting the heart disease of Covid-19: A systematic review

[117] Yang, L., Hou, A., et al. Panacis Quinquefolii Radix: A Review of the Botany, Phytochemistry, Quality Control, Pharmacology, Toxicology and Industrial Applications Research Progress

cognitive, anxiolytic and neuroprotective effects, which makes it a relevant choice for many long-Covid symptoms.[118]

Fu Shen (Poriae Cocos Pararadicis Sclerotium)

Fu Ling is an important herb for clearing dampness in the body. It tonifies the Spleen and calms the Heart. Fu Shen is the innermost part containing the root and it is specifically used for its spirit-calming effects.[119] This herb is important to use for any Gu patient exhibiting lingering dampness, loose stool and damaged Spleen Qi, as well as mental emotional, cognitive dysfunction, or insomnia.[120] It can help clear phlegm and thin mucus, aiding other herbs to penetrate into damp-phlegm biofilm where Gu pathogens may be residing. Poria has been seen to have some inhibitory effects on Covid-19.[121] Use it in any case where dampness and Spleen Qi deficiency are prominent.

---

[118] Szczuka, D., Nowak, A., et al. American Ginseng (Panax quinquefolium L.) as a Source of Bioactive Phytochemicals with Pro-Health Properties

[119] Bensky, et al. Materia Medica

[120] Sayed, S.E., Gomaa, S., et al. Sleep in post-Covid-19 recovery period and its impact on different domains of quality of life

[121] Wu, Z., Chen, X., et al. The inhibition of Mpro, the primary protease of Covid-19, by Poria cocos and its active compounds: a network pharmacology and molecular docking study

Tonify Qi and Blood with Pungent and Detoxifying Substances

Since Gu illnesses take a toll on the body's Qi and Yang Qi over time it was thought that pure tonic substances like Ren Shen (Asian Ginseng) can have the negative consequences of tonifying the Gu pathogen. For this reason, Gu formulas often contain tonic herbs which have the dual properties of being tonic as well as anti-parasitic.[122]

Huang Qi (Astragali Radix)

Huang Qi is an important tonic substance in the context of Covid-19 Gu Syndrome. It has the ability to tonify the Qi of both Lung and Spleen and it raises the Yang Qi. It is useful for symptoms of chronic fatigue, chronic low grade inflammation or

---

[122] Fruehauf, Heiner. Gu Syndrome: An In-depth Interview with Heiner Fruehauf

fever, immune deficiency, and shortness of breath.[123] It can reduce edema and benefits numb, weakened limb functions and painful obstruction. Combine it with Sheng Ma to lift sunken Qi.[124]

Huang Qi has important antiviral properties which are relevant for Covid-19 due to its immune modulating polysaccharides.[125] It is able to regulate the mucous membranes of the respiratory tract, which is a useful property for post-Covid patients with lingering Lung dysfunctions.[126] Importantly, it is also cardioprotective, and can help protect against viral induced myocarditis.[127] I think this may be an extremely important property to note in response to spike-induced myocardial damage.

---

[123] Bensky, et al. Materia Medica
[124] Ibid.
[125] Aleebrahim-Dehkordi, E., Heirdari-Soureshjani, E., et al. Antiviral Compounds Based on Natural Astragalus polysaccharides (APS): Research and Foresight in the Strategies for Combating SARS-CoV-2 (Covid-19)
[126] Lee, D.Y.W., Qing, Y.L., et al. Traditional Chinese herbal medicine at the forefront battle against Covid-19: Clinical experience and scientific basis
[127] Zheng, Q., Zhuang, Z., et al. Clinical and Preclinical Systematic Review of Astragalus Membranaceus for Viral Myocarditis

Dang Gui (Angelica Sinensis Radix)

Dang Gui is extremely pungent and it is a natural fit to both tonify blood deficiency and to move stagnant blood. It is often used for painful conditions and also to heal traumatic injury and regenerate tissues.[128] It is commonly paired with many other Gu herbs, making it a very flexible addition depending on the case. For example, it has been used as an adjunctive for cough, and can be paired with Zi Su Ye and Chen Pi. It has also been used to moisten the intestines in conjunction with He Shou Wu, or combined with Sheng Di Huang for blood deficiency. And it can be paired with Huang Qi for dual Qi and blood tonification.[129] Long-Covid syndrome does involve dysfunction of microcirculation and endothelial dysfunction.[130][131] Dang Gui is an herb which is used to promote and improve microcirculation, so one might also consider it as an herb in the invigorate stagnant Qi and Blood category as well.[132]

---

[128] Bensky, et al. Materia Medica

[129] Ibid.

[130] Charfeddine, S., et al. Long Covid 19 Syndrome: Is It Related to Microcirculation and Endothelial Dysfunction? Insights From TUN-EndCOV Study

[131] Zharkikh, E.V., et al. Assessment of Blood Microcirculation Changes after Covid-19 Using Wearable Laser Doppler Flowmetry

[132] Wu, Y., et al. Pharmacological effects of Radix Angelica Sinensis (Danggui) on cerebral infarction

Sheng He Shou Wu (Polygoni Multiflori Radix Non-preparata)

He Shou Wu in its unprocessed (sheng) form is mildly blood tonifying but also has an antimalarial, toxicity clearing action which the processed form does not have.[133] It moistens the intestines and is a mild laxative so it should not be used when patients have diarrhea; use it in ones with constipation.[134] It treats scrofula, sores, and toxic swellings, and can be combined with Xuan Shen and Lian Qiao for this.[135]

He Shou Wu has been found to inhibit the Covid-19 spike protein entry into cells.[136] He Shou Wu contains numerous phytochemicals, including phenols such as Catechin[137] and Gallic Acid.[138] Gallic Acid in particular has been shown to inhibit spike

---

[133] Bensky, et al. Materia Medica
[134] Fruehauf, Heiner. Gu Syndrome: An In-depth Interview with Heiner Fruehauf
[135] Bensky, et al. Materia Medica
[136] Wang, X., Lin, S., et al. Polygoni multiflori radix extracts inhibit SARS-CoV-2 pseudovirus entry in HEK293T cells and zebrafish larvae
[137] Arif, M.N. Catechin Derivatives as Inhibitor of Covid-19 Main Protease (Mpro): Molecular Docking Studies Unveil an Opportunity Against CORONA
[138] Liang, Z., Chen, H., et al. Comparison of raw and processed Radix Polygoni Multiflori (Heshouwu) by high performance liquid chromatography and mass spectrometry

protein entry at the receptor site.[139] Gallic Acid, and thus He Shou Wu, may be important therapeutics against Covid-19.[140]

Gan Cao (Radix Glycyrrhizae Uralensis)

Unprocessed raw Gan Cao, which has anti-toxin and antiparasitic properties, enters all twelve meridians but principally the Lung, Spleen, Heart, Stomach. It can also lead and conduct other herbs to meridians they wouldn't normally affect, making it an excellent envoy addition to formulas. Raw Gan Cao drains fire but with moderation, while also tonifying the Spleen Qi and moistening the Lungs.[141] Gan Cao should be included in Gu formulas for patients with a chronic, dry, lingering cough, or in deficiency patients with chronic fatigue or an irregular pulse. Sometimes it is paired with Bai Shao for spasms and muscle cramps, creating Shao Yao Gan Cao Tang.[142]

---

[139] Lin, S., Wang, X., et al. The Extracts of Polygonum cuspidatum Root and Rhizome Block the Entry of SARS-CoV-2 Wild-Type and Omicron Pseudotyped Viruses via Inhibition of the S-Protein and 3CL Protease

[140] Baraskar, K., Thakur, P., et al. Therapeutic Role of Phytophenol Gallic Acid for the Cure of Covid-19 Pathogenesis

[141] Bensky, et al. Materia Medica

[142] Ota, K. et al. Effect of Shakuyaku-kanzo-to in patients with muscle cramps: A systematic literature review

Gan Cao is known to have strong antiviral properties against many viruses[143], and this is true as well for Covid-19.[144] It has been considered as an auxiliary treatment for Covid.[145] In part, this is because of the anti-inflammatory, antiviral, and immunomodulatory effects of Glycyrrhizin, a prominent phytochemical in Licorice.[146] I think Gan Cao is a top tier herb to have in many long-haul Covid Gu Syndrome cases.

Bai Shao (Paeoniae Radix Alba)

Bai Shao softens the Liver, nourishes Blood, and extinguishes Wind. It is excellent at softening and nourishing the sinews, tonifying the Liver Blood, and extinguishing spasms.[147] It is commonly combined with Gan Cao to create Shao Yao Gan Cao Tang. It is also combined with Chai Hu and Dang Gui to be used in the formula Xiao Yao San for constrained Liver Qi with Blood

---

[143] Bailly, C., Vertogen, G. Glycyrrhizin: An alternative drug for the treatment of Covid-19 infection and the associated respiratory syndrome?

[144] Van de Sand, L., Bormann, L., et al. Glycyrrhizin Effectively Inhibits SARS-CoV-2 Replication by Inhibiting the Viral Main Protease

[145] Zhang, Q., Huang, H., et al. Traditional Uses, Pharmacological Effects, and Molecular Mechanisms of Licorice in Potential Therapy of Covid-19

[146] Chrzanowski, J., Chrzanowski, A., Grabon W. Glycyrrhizin: An old weapon against a novel coronavirus

[147] Bensky, et al. Materia Medica

stagnation.[148] Additionally, it can also be used with herbs like Sheng Di Huang to control internal Wind due to Yin deficiency.[149]

Bai Shao also has secondary Heart nourishing properties through its nourishing of Liver Blood.[150] Research suggests that Bai Shao has antidepressant effects.[151] It is also anti-inflammatory and immunomodulatory.[152] I would suggest this herb be added when patients exhibit symptoms of internal Wind, hyperactivity of the Liver, or depressive symptoms.

Wu Jia Pi (Eleutherococci Gracilistyli Cortex Radicis)

Wu Jia Pi is typically used for wind-damp painful Bi syndrome disorders such as pain in the joints and sinews, as it is good at unobstructing the free flow of Qi and Blood.[153] Dr. Heiner Fruehauf mentions that it is especially useful in Gu syndrome conditions when body pain is a main symptom, or when there are neurological or cognitive symptoms like brain fog, such as in

---

[148] Ibid.
[149] Ibid.
[150] Ibid.
[151] Mao, Q., Ip, S., et al. Anti-depressant-like effect of peony: a mini-review
[152] He, D., Dai, S. Anti-Inflammatory and Immunomodulatory Effects of Paeonia Lactiflora Pall., a Traditional Chinese Herbal Medicine
[153] Bensky, et al. Materia Medica

'Brain Gu'.[154] Adaptogenic herbs like Wu Jia Pi have many potentially beneficial effects on a number of dimensions for Covid long-haul patients, such as with pain, cognition, fatigue, and mood.[155]

---

[154] Fruehauf, Heiner. Gu Syndrome: An In-depth Interview with Heiner Fruehauf
[155] Karosanidze, I., Kiladze, U., et al. Efficacy of Adaptogens in Patients with Long Covid-19: A Randomized, Quadruple-Blind, Placebo-Controlled Trial

Invigorate Stagnant Qi and Blood to Expose Lingering Gu Pathogens

Covid-19 causes vascular endothelial damage and promotes platelet adhesion and coagulation, resulting in various forms of blood stagnation throughout the body and organs.[156] Promoting the movement of Qi and Blood is essential to driving out Gu pathogens which have 'set up shop' and ensconced themselves in hidden areas of the body, as well as to begin to heal and penetrate into the blood stagnation of damaged tissues, or where there is internal scarring. They also help to 'crack open' biofilms which may possibly be harboring viral particles.[157] This can assist the fumigative and antitoxin 'snake-killing' herbs

---

[156] Wang, C., Yu, C., et al. Long Covid: The Nature of Thrombotic Sequelae Determines the Necessity of Early Anticoagulation

[157] Von Borowski, R.G., Trentin, D.S. Biofilms and Coronavirus Reservoirs: a Perspective Review

to reach their targets.[158] In some cases the herbs in this category can bring symptomatic relief for painful conditions involving Qi and Blood stagnation.

Chen Pi (Citri Reticulatae Pericarpium)

Chen Pi is an aromatic herb which dries dampness and promotes the flow of Qi, particularly in the Stomach, Spleen, and Lungs. It helps to dry dampness and phlegm in the Lungs and Stomach with its aromatic nature, benefitting symptoms of chest and epigastric fullness, cough with sputum, abdominal distention, loose stool, belching, and nausea.[159] Pair it with Fu Ling to enhance the effects against damp-phlegm, or with Mu Xiang to settle stomach and abdominal fullness and pain. Chen Pi is also useful to help prevent stagnation and digestive bloating when used with other tonifying herbs.

As a citrus, Chen Pi also has a phytochemical called Hesperidin which has important neurological, cardiovascular, psychiatric, and anti-inflammatory effects.[160] Hesperidin has been studied for its potential inhibitory actions against Covid.[161]

---

[158] Fruehauf, Heiner. Gu Syndrome: An In-depth Interview with Heiner Fruehauf

[159] Bensky, et al. Materia Medica

[160] Li, C., Schluesener, H. Health-promoting effects of the citrus flavanone hesperidin

It has been recommended as both a prophylactic and a complementary therapy for Covid.[162]

Chai Hu (Bupleuri Radix)

Chai Hu is an aromatic herb which is prominently used to free constraint. It raises the Yang Qi, spreads Liver Qi, and expels constrained heat and pathogens trapped in the Shaoyang, providing a harmonizing action.[163] It can be combined with Dang Gui and Chuan Xiong to focus its harmonizing action on the blood.[164] It can be used as an auxiliary herb to help clear deficiency heat.[165]

Chai Hu has a number of biologically active phytochemicals which contribute to its anti-inflammatory, antiviral, and immunomodulatory actions.[166] Relevant phytochemicals with potentially therapeutic effects against Covid are the Saikosaponins contained in Chai Hu.[167]

---

[161] Cheng, F., Huynh, T., et al. Hesperidin Is a Potential Inhibitor against SARS-CoV-2 Infectio

[162] Bellavite, P., Dozelli, A. Hesperidin and SARS-CoV-2: New Light on the Healthy Function of Citrus Fruits

[163] Bensky, et al. Materia Medica

[164] Ibid.

[165] Ibid.

[166] Ashour, M.J., Wink, M. Genus Bupleurum: a review of its phytochemistry, pharmacology and modes of action

[167] Bahbah, E.I., Negida, A., Nabet, M.S. Purposing Saikosaponins for the treatment of Covid-19

Chuan Xiong (Chuan Xiong Rhizoma)

Chuan Xiong is used to invigorate the Qi and Blood and is helpful for conditions which involve blood stasis and wind. It is said to regulate the Qi within the Blood.[168] Chuan Xiong can be combined with Dang Gui, where Chuan Xiong enters the Qi aspect while Dang Gui enters the blood aspect, providing a synergistic broad-spectrum invigorating action.[169] Chuan Xiong can be used for many types of headache conditions. If a patient is blood deficient, it can combine with Bai Shao and Sheng Di Huang. Alternatively, it can be combined with herbs like Gao Ben for wind-damp disorders, or Chai Hu for when there is stagnation in the Liver and Shaoyang.[170]

Chuan Xiong is an herb which has commonly been used in treating plagues in China, and its polysaccharides have been considered for their potential against Covid-19.[171] It has been said to be an ideal therapeutic for treating cardiovascular and cerebrovascular issues due to its cardioprotective, anti-

---

[168] Bensky, et al. Materia Medica
[169] Ibid.
[170] Ibid.
[171] Wang, J., Wang, L., et al. The isolation, structural features and biological activities of polysaccharide from Ligusticum chuanxiong: A review

hypertensive, anti-inflammatory, and anti-thrombotic properties.[172] Research suggests it also has neuroprotective properties and can protect against cerebral ischemia and helps promote neurogenesis and reduce inflammation.[173] Due to these properties, it should be considered in many Heart and Brain Gu disorders, and in formulas where invigorating the Qi and Blood is a general goal.

Mu Xiang (Aucklandiae Radix)

Mu Xiang, which translates literally as 'wood fragrance', is a warming and aromatic Qi regulating herb which focuses its actions on the digestive organs and the Shaoyang. It is commonly used for digestive disorders such as diarrhea, tenesmus, abdominal pain, nausea, distention, or digestive stagnation. It can help clear damp-heat, ameliorate digestive side effects of tonification herbs on the Stomach, as well as aid anti-parasitic herbs focusing on the intestines.[174] Add it in formulas for Gu patients who have a sensitive digestion, or who present with Digestive Gu.

---

[172] Chen, Z., Zhang, C., et al. A systematic review on the rhizome of Ligusticum chuanxiong Hort. (Chuanxiong)

[173] Wang, M., Yao, M., et al. Ligusticum chuanxiong exerts neuroprotection by promoting adult neurogenesis and inhibiting inflammation in the hippocampus of ME cerebral ischemia rats

[174] Bensky, et al. Materia Medica

E Zhu (Curcumae Rhizoma)

E Zhu is used to forcefully break up blood stagnation and blood stasis, promote the movement of Qi and Blood, dissolve masses, as well as resolve food stagnation and phlegm.[175] These qualities make it important in the context of hidden pathogens lurking enclosed within phlegm, biofilms, and stagnant tissues. It can be combined with other Gu herbs such as Mu Xiang for food stagnation, or other blood stasis breaking herbs such as San Leng. Comparatively, E Zhu focuses more on Qi stagnation than San Leng, which has more focused action on breaking up stagnant blood.[176] E Zhu 'grinds away' at masses and accumulations, and it, too, has an aromatic quality useful for Gu Syndrome.[177]

This is definitely an important herb in the context of Covid. Curcumin was one of the first phytochemicals studied for potential activity against Covid, early in the pandemic.[178] It has also been suggested as a prophylactic therapy for Covid.[179] Some

---

[175] Ibid.
[176] Ibid.
[177] Ibid.
[178] Rajagopal, K., Varakumar, P., et al. Activity of phytochemical constituents of Curcuma longa (turmeric) and Andrographis paniculata against coronavirus (Covid-19): an in silico approach
[179] Thimmulappa, R.K., Mudnakudu-Nagaraju, K.K., et al. Antiviral and immunomodulatory activity of curcumin: A case for prophylactic

have even called it a 'wonder drug' in the prevention of Covid.[180] I think Curcumae herbal variants have a place in almost any Covid Gu formula due to them being rich in the phytochemical curcumin.[181]

San Leng (Sparganii Rhizoma)

San Leng pairs well with E Zhu, but focuses more strongly on breaking up and cracking open Blood stagnation and dissolving lumps, masses, and stagnant clumping. It is a fairly strong natured herb in this respect and extra caution might be used with patients prone to bleeding disorders.[182]

San Qi (Notoginseng Radix)

San Qi is an herb which is used to prevent bleeding but simultaneously transform blood stasis, making it extremely functionally useful. It is used for many types of traumatic injuries and for stopping pain, including chest, abdominal, and

---

therapy for Covid-19

[180] Manoharan, Y., Haridas, V., et al. Curcumin: a Wonder Drug as a Preventive Measure for Covid19 Management

[181] Vahedian-Azimi, A., Abbasifard, M., et al. Effectiveness of Curcumin on Outcomes of Hospitalized Covid-19 Patients: A Systematic Review of Clinical Trials

[182] Bensky, et al. Materia Medica

joint pains which involve blood stasis.[183] This is an important herb for its blood regulating powers.

It has also been studied for its uses in numerous conditions such as coronary heart disease,[184] angina pectoris[185], cerebral ischemia,[186] and a variety of inflammation-related chronic diseases, many of which overlap with long-Covid symptomatologies.[187] It has also been studied for its neuroprotective, anxiolytic and antidepressant effects. Some of its biological activity can be partially explained by its Saponin content.[188] I believe this is an important and useful herb to combine with other blood stasis herbs for Covid Gu formulas.

---

[183] Ibid.

[184] Shang, Q., Xu, H., et al. Oral Panax notoginseng Preparation for Coronary Heart Disease: A Systematic Review of Randomized Controlled Trials

[185] Song, H., Wang, P., et al. Panax notoginseng Preparations for Unstable Angina Pectoris: A Systematic Review and Meta-Analysis

[186] Yang, F., Ma, Q., et al. Panax notoginseng for Cerebral Ischemia: A Systematic Review

[187] Xu, Y., Tan, H., et al. Panax notoginseng for Inflammation-Related Chronic Diseases: A Review on the Modulations of Multiple Pathways

[188] Xie, W., Meng, X., et al. Panax Notoginseng Saponins: A Review of Its Mechanisms of Antidepressant or Anxiolytic Effects and Network Analysis on Phytochemistry and Pharmacology

Ze Lan (Lycopi Herba)

Ze Lan focuses on invigorating the blood in a harmonious and gentle way, while also promoting urination. Perhaps one reason it is used in Gu formulas is that its aromatic nature "pierces congealed Yin."[189] Its ability to promote urination makes it an ideal selection in patients who are harboring water accumulation and have edema, such as facial edema or edema in the extremities.[190]

Bai Guo Ye (Ginkgo Folium)

Bai Guo Ye may be a useful herb in the context of Covid Gu Syndrome. Traditionally, it is used to arrest wheezing and coughing with sputum, as well as having a blood invigorating action.[191] The leaves of the Ginkgo plant were used more in western herbalism than in Chinese traditional medicine. However its antiviral activities have made Ginkgo an herb recommended for further study with relation to Covid.[192] It has been noted to exhibit pulmonary protective, anti-inflammatory

---

[189] Bensky, et al. Materia Medica
[190] Ibid.
[191] Ibid.
[192] Ibrahim, M.A., Ramadan, H.H., Mohammed, R.N. Evidence that Ginkgo Biloba could use in the influenza and coronavirus Covid-19 infections

and anti-thrombotic properties, and some have recommended it as a complement to Covid treatment.[193] It has also been studied in the context of cognitive impairment and dementia.[194] It is thought to have memory enhancing effects.[195] This is perhaps due to its ability to increase cerebral blood flow,[196] which is something that may be useful in the context of the brain fog experienced by Covid patients and the known ability of the spike protein to cross the blood-brain barrier and cause potential damage.

---

[193] Al-Kuraishy, H.M., Al-Gareeb, A.I., et al. Ginkgo biloba in the management of the Covid-19 severity

[194] Zhang, H., Huang., L., et al. An Overview of Systematic Reviews of Ginkgo biloba Extracts for Mild Cognitive Impairment and Dementia

[195] Field, B.H., Vadnal, R. Ginkgo biloba and Memory: An Overview

[196] Mashayekh, A., Pham, D.L., et al. Effects of Ginkgo biloba on cerebral blood flow assessed by quantitative MR perfusion imaging: a pilot study

Su He Tang:
A Basis for Modified Gu Formulas

Formula: Su He Tang (Perilla and Mint Decoction)[197]

Source: Lu Shunde, Zhi Gu Xinfang (New Methods for the Treatment of Gu Syndrome), Qing Dynasty.

Indications: treats all types of Gu syndrome including various expressions of 'snake Gu' and 'emaciation Gu', and Gu related disorders involving bloating, swelling, madness, depression and epilepsy. Secondary symptoms include 'flu-like symptoms, coughing or other signs of Qi counterflow, or a tight abdominal wall. Generally it can be said that this decoction is designed for Gu syndrome involving the internal sweltering of excess fire

---

[197] Fruehauf, H. Traditional Chinese Approaches to Gu Syndrome: Two 18th Century Examples

(important signs: dark urine, patient usually gets worse after ingesting tonics).

Ingredients and Administration:

Bo He (Herba Menthae) 30g

Zi Su Ye (Folium Perillae Frutescentis) 30g

Tiao Shen/ Bei Sha Shen (Radix Glehniae Littoralis) 24g

Lian Qiao (Fructus Forsythiae Suspensae) 24g

Huang Qi (Radix Astragali) 21g

Dang Gui (Radix Angelicae Sinensis) 30g

Sheng He Shou Wu (Unprocessed Radix Polygoni Multiflori) 30g

Bai Zhi (Radix Angelicae) 30g

Chuan Xiong (Radix Ligustici Wallichii) 15g

Jue Ming Zi (Semen Cassiae Torae) 15g

Huai Hua (Flos Sophorae Japonicae Immaturus) 30g

Bai Shao (Radix Paeoniae Lactiflorae) 15g

Chai Hu (Radix Bupleuri) 18g

Qing Hao (Herba Artemisiae Apiaceae) 30g

Sheng Yuanban/Sheng Di Huang (Radix Rehmanniae Glutinosae) 24g

Decoct in water. If San Qi (Radix Notoginseng) 6g is added, the results will be enhanced.

Su He Tang (Perilla and Mint Decoction)

Su He Tang (and its modified version Jia Jian Su He Tang) is a Qing Dynasty formula for Gu Syndrome which has served as a basis for modern variations such as Lightning and Thunder Pearls, developed by Dr. Heiner Fruehauf and distributed by Classical Pearls.[198][199] On Su He Tang, Dr. Fruehauf says: "I picked two formulas that did not contain any exotic or toxic substances for the purpose of clinical experimentation: Su He Tang (Perilla and Mint Decoction) and Jiajian Su He Tang (Modified Perilla and Mint Decoction), both recorded in the Qing dynasty work Zhigu xinfang (New Formulas for the Treatment of Gu). All herbs in these formulas are easily recognizable, and together present an understandable approach of tonifying deficiency, eliminating wind and damp influences, killing parasitic toxins directly, and at the same time reducing ancillary symptoms like anxiety. This method made sense to me, so during the last 20 years I have stuck with modifications of this remedy."[200]

---

[198] Classical Pearls

[199] I am not associated with Classical Pearls or Dr. Fruehauf, but I have used these two products with moderate success in various long-Covid and Gu Syndrome cases.

[200] Fruehauf, H.. An Ancient Solution for Modern Diseases: "Gu Syndrome" and Chronic Inflammatory Diseases with Autoimmune Complications (An Interview with Heiner Fruehauf)

I agree with his strategy and think that other variations can also be made specific to individual manifestations of long-haul Covid-19 Gu Syndrome. For example, I think formulas which take into account whether the constellation of post-Covid symptoms are primarily Pulmonary, Circulatory, Neurologically, etc. and modified accordingly, will be most effective. A systems-centered approach can guide and focus a custom herbal formula and treatment plan similar to how Brain or Digestive Gu are differentiated in Lightning and Thunder Pearls.

Modifications for Covid Lung & Heart Gu

Appropriate modifications should be made according to the symptoms and differential diagnosis of each individual patient. Using Su He Tang as a base, we can choose modifications from the most appropriate herbs in the list overviewed above, as well as by exercising our normal pattern discrimination and diagnostic herbal medicine skills. There may indeed be other herbs not included in this document but which may also be useful which lie outside the scope of this analysis. The following chart is an example of herbs which may be relevant specifically to Lung and Heart Gu Syndromes.

Lung Gu Formula Example	Heart Gu Formula Example
Zi Su Ye Bo He Bai Zhi Jin Yin Hua Huang Qi Ding Xiang He Zi Bai He Sha Shen Xuan Shen Huang Qi Gan Cao Chen Pi	Zi Su Ye Jin Yin Hua Lian Qiao Tulsi Da Suan / Garlic E Zhu San Qi Dang Gui Chen Pi Chuan Xiong Ze Lan Xi Yang Shen Bai Shao Huang Qi Sheng Di Huang Gan Cao

Note: These formulations and modifications are theoretical examples; herbalists should develop custom formulas for individual cases based on the many factors involved. One must also take into account contraindications such as herb-drug interactions when selecting herbs.

Dosage:

Another aspect of treatment relayed by Dr. Fruehauf is the usefulness of starting with small dosages and slowly working up to full dosage in order to avoid triggering an overactive acute immune reaction. He states that: "Often these type of patients have many symptoms because they tend to be allergic. Both the Brain Gu type as well as the Digestive Gu type can exhibit many auto-immune symptoms, including food allergies, and often react extremely sensitively to stimuli in their environment. It is important, therefore, that you work your way up to the target amount slowly. These patients can react poorly to herbs, even if it is the right formula, if you dose initially too high. It is better to start on the low end and work your way up to the medium or high range."[201] Part of this may be related to his recognition that, as opposed to environmental toxins, "Living pathogens, will employ sophisticated evasion strategies once they feel attacked."[202] Especially in cases involving the heart and circulatory system one should exercise caution. It is important to avoid possible adverse herb-drug interactions.

Administration:

Dr. Fruehauf notes that alongside the chronic heat and inflammation which accompanies autoimmune Gu diseases comes severe chronic deficiency as well, so it can be helpful to note that he eventually recommends Yang tonification after the

---

[201] Ibid.
[202] Fruehauf, Heiner. Gu Syndrome: An In-depth Interview with Heiner Fruehauf

first stages of Gu treatment. "The more inflamed someone is, the more energy is lost over time. So, depending on their degree of yang deficiency, you have to give them serious yang tonics such as Sini Tang along with the Gu herbs, either right away in very cold patients, or after six months when the body is asking to switch to recharge mode in most patients. This is the only effective way to contain and gradually repair the trauma in their immune system."[203]

During the course of treatment, the formula can be continually modified with herbs from the list such as by switching out one herb from each category. "Since we are dealing with a living pathogen that has the ability to adapt, I recommend a regular change in the details of the prescription. It is best to change a Gu prescription regimen, at least somewhat, every six weeks. The classical record already points this out, by warning about the ability of Gu pathogens to adapt, and suggesting to always stay a step ahead by making changes to your herbal approach. Changing the formula means that you leave the six categories intact—those categories never change, they are in every Gu formula— but of the two or three herbs in a particular category you always rotate at least one out and put a new one from the same category in. In this way, the general

---

[203] Ibid.

arrow of the therapeutic approach never changes, but you change the herbs within it."[204]

When the chronic pathogens have been cleared, it is time to cease administering Gu formulas and begin a process of tonification, such as with Yang tonics or other medicinals as necessary according to individual pattern discrimination and diagnostics.

---

[204] Fruehauf, H.. An Ancient Solution for Modern Diseases: "Gu Syndrome" and Chronic Inflammatory Diseases with Autoimmune Complications (An Interview with Heiner Fruehauf)

Conclusion

The scientific literature describes some of the current understanding about persistent viral pathogens, chronic disease, and long term health. There is a paucity of support and treatment options for patients suffering from long-covid symptoms and pathologies, leading to many seeking out alternatives.[205]

Many symptoms of long-haul Covid resonate with the ancient concept of chronic Gu Syndrome and its modern interpretations by scholar-practitioners. Gu Syndrome therefore represents a potentially useful clinical lens through which we can view long-haul Covid-19 from our medical tradition. It can provide a conceptual and theoretical framework for devising new herbal formulations and treatment strategies for this novel disease.

We have seen that in many cases the herbs used in classical Gu Syndrome formulas have at least some scientific evidence for their inhibitory actions against Covid-19 and/or potential therapeutic effects. Gu treatment strategies are flexible and can be modified to fit the specific manifestations of long-haul Covid patients and their individual symptoms and differential

---

[205] Brown, L., et al. Long COVID and self-management

diagnoses for greatest effectiveness. Consider using this guide as an evolving framework for constructing individualized herbal formulations for long-Covid Gu Syndromes.

References

Abrahim, M.A.A., Mohamed, E.A.R., et al. Rutin and flavone analogs as prospective SARS-CoV-2 main protease inhibitors: In silico drug discovery study. J Mol Graph Model. 2021 Jun;105:107904. doi: 10.1016/j.jmgm.2021.107904. Epub 2021 Mar 20. https://pubmed.ncbi.nlm.nih.gov/33798836/

Agrawal, P.K., Agrawal, C., Blunden, G. Artemisia Extracts and Artemisinin-Based Antimalarials for Covid-19 Management: Could These Be Effective Antivirals for Covid-19 Treatment? Molecules. 2022 Jun; 27(12): 3828. Published online 2022 Jun 14. doi: 10.3390/molecules27123828. https://www.ncbi.nlm.nih.gov/pmc/articles/PMC9231170/

Al-Kuraishy, H.M., Al-Gareeb, A.I., et al. Ginkgo biloba in the management of the Covid-19 severity. Arch Pharm (Weinheim). 2022 Oct;355(10):e2200188. doi: 10.1002/ardp.202200188. Epub 2022 Jun 7. https://pubmed.ncbi.nlm.nih.gov/35672257/

Al-Kuraishy, H.M., Al-Gareeb, A.I., et al. The possible role of ursolic acid in Covid-19: A real game changer. Clin Nutr ESPEN. 2022 Feb;47:414-417. doi: 10.1016/j.clnesp.2021.12.030. Epub 2022 Jan 4. https://pubmed.ncbi.nlm.nih.gov/35063236/

Aleebrahim-Dehkordi, E., Heirdari-Soureshjani, E., et al. Antiviral Compounds Based on Natural Astragalus polysaccharides (APS): Research and Foresight in the Strategies for Combating SARS-CoV-2 (Covid-19). Mini Rev Med Chem. 2022;22(17):2299-2307. doi: 10.2174/1389557522666220301143113. https://pubmed.ncbi.nlm.nih.gov/35232341/

Almehdi, A., Khoder, G., et al. SARS-CoV-2 spike protein: pathogenesis, vaccines, and potential therapies. Infection. 2021; 49(5): 855–876. Published online 2021 Aug 2. doi: 10.1007/s15010-021-01677-8. https://www.ncbi.nlm.nih.gov/pmc/articles/PMC8326314/

Arif, M.N. Catechin Derivatives as Inhibitor of Covid-19 Main Protease (Mpro): Molecular Docking Studies Unveil an Opportunity Against CORONA. Comb Chem High Throughput Screen. 2022;25(1):197-203. doi:

10.2174/1871520620666201123101002. https://pubmed.ncbi.nlm.nih.gov/33231155/

Ashour, M.J., Wink, M. Genus Bupleurum: a review of its phytochemistry, pharmacology and modes of action. J Pharm Pharmacol. 2011 Mar;63(3):305-21. doi: 10.1111/j.2042-7158.2010.01170.x. Epub 2010 Nov 16. https://pubmed.ncbi.nlm.nih.gov/21749378/

Aucott, J.N., Rebman, A.W. Long-haul Covid: heed the lessons from other infection-triggered illnesses. Lancet. 2021 13-19 March; 397(10278): 967–968. Published online 2021 Mar 5. doi: 10.1016/S0140-6736(21)00446-3. https://www.ncbi.nlm.nih.gov/pmc/articles/PMC7952095/

Bailly, C., Vertogen, G. Glycyrrhizin: An alternative drug for the treatment of Covid-19 infection and the associated respiratory syndrome? Pharmacol Ther. 2020 Oct; 214: 107618. Published online 2020 Jun 24. doi: 10.1016/j.pharmthera.2020.107618. https://www.ncbi.nlm.nih.gov/pmc/articles/PMC7311916/

Bahbah, E.I., Negida, A., Nabet, M.S. Purposing Saikosaponins for the treatment of Covid-19. Med Hypotheses. 2020 Jul; 140: 109782. Published online 2020 Apr 23. doi: 10.1016/j.mehy.2020.109782. https://www.ncbi.nlm.nih.gov/pmc/articles/PMC7179490/

Banerjee, S., Wang, X., et al. Comprehensive role of SARS-CoV-2 spike glycoprotein in regulating host signaling pathway. J Med Virol. 2022 Sep;94(9):4071-4087. doi: 10.1002/jmv.27820. Epub 2022 May 9. https://pubmed.ncbi.nlm.nih.gov/35488404/

Bansal, A.S., Bradley, A.A., et al. Chronic fatigue syndrome, the immune system and viral infection. Brain Behav Immun. 2012 Jan;26(1):24-31. doi: 10.1016/j.bbi.2011.06.016. Epub 2011 Jul 2. https://pubmed.ncbi.nlm.nih.gov/21756995/

Baraskar, K., Thakur, P., et al. Therapeutic Role of Phytophenol Gallic Acid for the Cure of Covid-19 Pathogenesis. Endocr Metab Immune Disord Drug Targets. 2022 Aug 29. doi: 10.2174/1871530322666220829141401. Online ahead of print. https://pubmed.ncbi.nlm.nih.gov/36043737/

Bellanti, J.A. The long Covid syndrome: A conundrum for the allergist/immunologist. Allergy Asthma Proc. 2022 Sep; 43(5): 368–374. doi: 10.2500/aap.2022.43.220059. https://www.ncbi.nlm.nih.gov/pmc/articles/PMC9465643/

Bellavite, P., Dozelli, A. Hesperidin and SARS-CoV-2: New Light on the Healthy Function of Citrus Fruits. Antioxidants (Basel). 2020 Aug; 9(8): 742. Published online 2020 Aug 13. doi: 10.3390/antiox9080742. https://www.ncbi.nlm.nih.gov/pmc/articles/PMC7465267/

Bensky, D., Clavey, S., et al. Chinese Herbal Medicine Materia Medica 3rd Ed. Eastland Pr; 3rd edition (September 1, 2004). ISBN-10 : 0939616424

Bogariu, A.M., Dumitrascu, D.L. Digestive involvement in the Long-Covid syndrome. Med Pharm Rep. 2022 Jan; 95(1): 5–10. Published online 2022 Jan 31. doi: 10.15386/mpr-2340. https://www.ncbi.nlm.nih.gov/pmc/articles/PMC9177081/

Brown, J.J., et al. A viral trigger for celiac disease. PLoS Pathog. 2018 Sep; 14(9): e1007181.Published online 2018 Sep 20. doi: 10.1371/journal.ppat.1007181. https://www.ncbi.nlm.nih.gov/pmc/articles/PMC6147651/

Brown, L., et al. Long COVID and self-management. Lancet. 2022 22-28 January; 399(10322): 355. Published online 2022 Jan 20. doi: 10.1016/S0140-6736(21)02798-7

Cai, B., Zhang, Y., et al. Therapeutic Potential of Diosgenin and Its Major Derivatives against Neurological Diseases: Recent Advances. Oxid Med Cell Longev. 2020; 2020: 3153082. Published online 2020 Mar 6. doi: 10.1155/2020/3153082. https://www.ncbi.nlm.nih.gov/pmc/articles/PMC7079249/

Charfeddine, S., et al. Long Covid 19 Syndrome: Is It Related to Microcirculation and Endothelial Dysfunction? Insights From TUN-EndCOV Study. Front Cardiovasc Med. 2021 Nov 30:8:745758. doi: 10.3389/fcvm.2021.745758. eCollection 2021.

Chen, Z., Zhang, C., et al. A systematic review on the rhizome of Ligusticum chuanxiong Hort. (Chuanxiong). Food Chem Toxicol. 2018 Sep;119:309-325. doi: 10.1016/j.fct.2018.02.050. Epub 2018 Feb 24. https://pubmed.ncbi.nlm.nih.gov/29486278/

Cheng, F., Huynh, T., et al. Hesperidin Is a Potential Inhibitor against SARS-CoV-2 Infection. Nutrients. 2021 Aug 16;13(8):2800. doi: 10.3390/nu13082800. https://pubmed.ncbi.nlm.nih.gov/34444960/

Chhabra, N., Grill, M.F., Singh, R.B.H. Post-Covid Headache: A Literature Review. Curr Pain Headache Rep. 2022; 26(11): 835–842. Published online 2022 Oct 5. doi: 10.1007/s11916-022-01086-y. https://www.ncbi.nlm.nih.gov/pmc/articles/PMC9533267/

Chrzanowski, J., Chrzanowski, A., Grabon W. Glycyrrhizin: An old weapon against a novel coronavirus. Phytother Res. 2021 Feb;35(2):629-636. doi: 10.1002/ptr.6852. Epub 2020 Sep 9. https://pubmed.ncbi.nlm.nih.gov/32902005/

Classical Pearls. https://www.classicalpearls.org/

Cohen, M.M. Tulsi - Ocimum sanctum: A herb for all reasons. J Ayurveda Integr Med. 2014 Oct-Dec; 5(4): 251–259. doi: 10.4103/0975-9476.146554. https://www.ncbi.nlm.nih.gov/pmc/articles/PMC4296439/

Cosentino, M., Marino, F. Understanding the Pharmacology of Covid-19 mRNA Vaccines: Playing Dice with the Spike? Int J Mol Sci. 2022 Sep 17;23(18):10881. doi: 10.3390/ijms231810881.

DeOre, B.J., Tran, K.A., et al. SARS-CoV-2 Spike Protein Disrupts Blood-Brain Barrier Integrity via RhoA Activation. J Neuroimmune Pharmacol. 2021 Dec;16(4):722-728. doi: 10.1007/s11481-021-10029-0. Epub 2021 Oct 23. https://pubmed.ncbi.nlm.nih.gov/34687399/

Donma, M.M., Donma, O. The effects of allium sativum on immunity within the scope of Covid-19 infection. Med Hypotheses. 2020 Nov;144:109934. doi: 10.1016/j.mehy.2020.109934. Epub 2020 Jun 2. https://pubmed.ncbi.nlm.nih.gov/32512493/

Erickson, M.A., Rhea, E.M., et al. Interactions of SARS-CoV-2 with the Blood–Brain Barrier. Int J Mol Sci. 2021 Mar; 22(5): 2681. Published online 2021 Mar 6. doi: 10.3390/ijms22052681. https://www.ncbi.nlm.nih.gov/pmc/articles/PMC7961671/

Faksova, A., et al. COVID-19 vaccines and adverse events of special interest: A multinational Global Vaccine Data Network (GVDN) cohort study of 99 million vaccinated individuals

Field, B.H., Vadnal, R. Ginkgo biloba and Memory: An Overview. Nutr Neurosci. 1998;1(4):255-67. doi: 10.1080/1028415X.1998.11747236. https://pubmed.ncbi.nlm.nih.gov/27414695/

Firaz, A., et al. Covid-19 and retinal degenerative diseases: Promising link "Kaempferol". Curr Opin Pharmacol. 2022 Jun; 64: 102231. Published online 2022 Apr 14. doi: 10.1016/j.coph.2022.102231

Fruehauf, Heiner. An Ancient Solution for Modern Diseases: "Gu Syndrome" and Chronic Inflammatory Diseases with Autoimmune Complications (An Interview with Heiner Fruehauf). https://classicalchinesemedicine.org/heiner-fruehauf-gu-syndrome-chronic-inflammation-autoimmune/

Fruehauf, Heiner. Driving Out Demons and Snakes: A Forgotten Clinical Approach to Chronic Parasitism. Classical Chinese Medicine. The Journal of Chinese Medicine (Issue 57). May 1998. https://www.journalofchinesemedicine.com/the-journal/jcm-article-archive/acupuncture-techniques/miscellaneous-442/driving-out-demons-and-snakes-gu-syndrome-and-a-forgotten-clinical-approach-to-chronic-parasitism.html

Fruehauf, Heiner. Gu Syndrome: An In-depth Interview with Heiner Fruehauf. https://classicalchinesemedicine.org/gu-syndrome-interview-heiner-fruehauf/

Fruehauf, Heiner. Traditional Chinese Approaches to Gu Syndrome: Two 18th Century Examples. 2011. https://classicalchinesemedicine.org/wp-content/uploads/2012/01/fruehauf_guapproaches.pdf

Fuzimoto, A.D. An overview of the anti-SARS-CoV-2 properties of Artemisia annua, its antiviral action, protein-associated mechanisms, and repurposing for Covid-19 treatment. J Integr Med. 2021 Sep;19(5):375-388. doi: 10.1016/j.joim.2021.07.003. Epub 2021 Jul 22. https://pubmed.ncbi.nlm.nih.gov/34479848/

Grigoriadis, N., Hadjigeorgiou, G.M. Virus-mediated autoimmunity in Multiple Sclerosis. J Autoimmune Dis. 2006; 3: 1. Published online 2006 Feb 19. doi: 10.1186/1740-2557-3-1. https://www.ncbi.nlm.nih.gov/pmc/articles/PMC1397830/

Gu (poison). Wikipedia. https://en.wikipedia.org/wiki/Gu_(poison)

He, D., Dai, S. Anti-Inflammatory and Immunomodulatory Effects of Paeonia Lactiflora Pall., a Traditional Chinese Herbal Medicine. Front Pharmacol. 2011; 2: 10. Published online 2011 Feb 25. doi: 10.3389/fphar.2011.00010. https://www.ncbi.nlm.nih.gov/pmc/articles/PMC3108611/

Hossain, M.A., Kim, J. Possibility as role of ginseng and ginsenosides on inhibiting the heart disease of Covid-19: A systematic review. J Ginseng Res. 2022 May;46(3):321-330. doi: 10.1016/j.jgr.2022.01.003. Epub 2022 Jan 19. https://pubmed.ncbi.nlm.nih.gov/35068945/

Ibrahim, M.A., Ramadan, H.H., Mohammed, R.N. Evidence that Ginkgo Biloba could use in the influenza and coronavirus Covid-19 infections. J Basic Clin Physiol Pharmacol. 2021 Feb 16;32(3):131-143. doi: 10.1515/jbcpp-2020-0310.https://pubmed.ncbi.nlm.nih.gov/33559843/

Imig, J.D. SARS-CoV-2 spike protein causes cardiovascular disease independent of viral infection. Clin Sci (Lond). 2022 Mar; 136(6): 431–434. Published online 2022 Mar 29. doi: 10.1042/CS20220028

Karosanidze, I., Kiladze, U., et al. Efficacy of Adaptogens in Patients with Long Covid-19: A Randomized, Quadruple-Blind, Placebo-Controlled Trial. Pharmaceuticals (Basel). 2022 Mar; 15(3): 345. Published online 2022 Mar 11. doi: 10.3390/ph15030345. https://www.ncbi.nlm.nih.gov/pmc/articles/PMC8953947/

Kartsoli, S., Vrakas, S., et al. Ulcerative colitis after SARS-CoV-2 infection. Autops Case Rep. 2022; 12: e2021378. Published online 2022 Apr 28. doi: 10.4322/acr.2021.378. https://www.ncbi.nlm.nih.gov/pmc/articles/PMC9083785/

Khubber, S., Hashemifesharaki, R., et al. Garlic (Allium sativum L.): a potential unique therapeutic food rich in organosulfur and flavonoid compounds to fight with Covid-19. Nutr J. 2020; 19: 124. Published online 2020 Nov 18. doi: 10.1186/s12937-020-00643-8. https://www.ncbi.nlm.nih.gov/pmc/articles/PMC7673072/

Lam, K.Y.C., Chen, J., et al. Asarone from Acori Tatarinowii Rhizoma Potentiates the Nerve Growth Factor-Induced Neuronal Differentiation in Cultured PC12 Cells: A Signaling Mediated by Protein Kinase A. PLoS One. 2016; 11(9): e0163337. Published online 2016 Sep 29. doi: 10.1371/journal.pone.0163337. https://www.ncbi.nlm.nih.gov/pmc/articles/PMC5042514/

Lee, B.W., Ha, T.K.Q., et al. Antiviral activity of furanocoumarins isolated from Angelica dahurica against influenza a viruses H1N1 and H9N2. J Ethnopharmacol. 2020 Sep 15;259:112945. doi: 10.1016/j.jep.2020.112945. Epub 2020 May 7. https://pubmed.ncbi.nlm.nih.gov/32389854/

Lee, D.Y.W., Qing, Y.L., et al. Traditional Chinese herbal medicine at the forefront battle against Covid-19: Clinical experience and scientific basis. Phytomedicine. 2021 Jan; 80: 153337. Published online 2020 Sep 28. doi: 10.1016/j.phymed.2020.153337. https://www.ncbi.nlm.nih.gov/pmc/articles/PMC7521884/

Lee, H., Kim, H., et al. Scrophulariae Radix: An Overview of Its Biological Activities and Nutraceutical and Pharmaceutical Applications. Molecules. 2021 Sep; 26(17): 5250. Published online 2021 Aug 30. doi: 10.3390/molecules26175250. https://www.ncbi.nlm.nih.gov/pmc/articles/PMC8434300/

Li, C., Schluesener, H. Health-promoting effects of the citrus flavanone hesperidin. Crit Rev Food Sci Nutr. 2017 Feb 11;57(3):613-631. doi: 10.1080/10408398.2014.906382.
https://pubmed.ncbi.nlm.nih.gov/25675136/

Liang, Z., Chen, H., et al. Comparison of raw and processed Radix Polygoni Multiflori (Heshouwu) by high performance liquid chromatography and mass spectrometry. Chin Med. 2010; 5: 29. Published online 2010 Aug 12. doi: 10.1186/1749-8546-5-29.
https://www.ncbi.nlm.nih.gov/pmc/articles/PMC2930642/

Lin, H., Wang, X., et al. Exploring the treatment of Covid-19 with Yinqiao powder based on network pharmacology. Phytother Res. 2021 May; 35(5): 2651–2664. Published online 2021 Jan 15. doi: 10.1002/ptr.7012.
https://www.ncbi.nlm.nih.gov/pmc/articles/PMC8013442/

Lin, S., Wang, X., et al. The Extracts of Polygonum cuspidatum Root and Rhizome Block the Entry of SARS-CoV-2 Wild-Type and Omicron Pseudotyped Viruses via Inhibition of the S-Protein and 3CL Protease. Molecules. 2022 Jun; 27(12): 3806. Published online 2022 Jun 13. doi: 10.3390/molecules27123806.
https://www.ncbi.nlm.nih.gov/pmc/articles/PMC9231230/

Liu, F., Zhao, Q., et al. Revealing the Pharmacological Mechanism of Acorus tatarinowii in the Treatment of Ischemic Stroke Based on Network Pharmacology. Evid Based Complement Alternat Med. 2020 Oct 31;2020:3236768. doi: 10.1155/2020/3236768. eCollection 2020.
https://pubmed.ncbi.nlm.nih.gov/33178313/

Maltezou, H.Z., Pavli, A., Tsakris, A. Post-Covid Syndrome: An Insight on Its Pathogenesis. Vaccines (Basel). 2021 May; 9(5): 497. Published online 2021 May 12. doi: 10.3390/vaccines9050497.
https://www.ncbi.nlm.nih.gov/pmc/articles/PMC8151752/

Manoharan, Y., Haridas, V., et al. Curcumin: a Wonder Drug as a Preventive Measure for Covid19 Management. Indian J Clin Biochem. 2020 Jul; 35(3): 373–375. Published online 2020 Jun 17. doi: 10.1007/s12291-020-00902-9.
https://www.ncbi.nlm.nih.gov/pmc/articles/PMC7299138/

Mao, Q., Ip, S., et al. Anti-depressant-like effect of peony: a mini-review. Pharm Biol. 2012 Jan;50(1):72-7. doi: 10.3109/13880209.2011.602696.
https://pubmed.ncbi.nlm.nih.gov/22196583/

Mashayekh, A., Pham, D.L., et al. Effects of Ginkgo biloba on cerebral blood flow assessed by quantitative MR perfusion imaging: a pilot study.

Neuroradiology. 2011 Mar;53(3):185-91. doi: 10.1007/s00234-010-0790-6. https://pubmed.ncbi.nlm.nih.gov/21061003/

Maurya, R., Sebastian, P., et al. Covid-19 Severity in Obesity: Leptin and Inflammatory Cytokine Interplay in the Link Between High Morbidity and Mortality. Front Immunol. 2021; 12: 649359. Published online 2021 Jun 18. doi: 10.3389/fimmu.2021.649359. https://www.ncbi.nlm.nih.gov/pmc/articles/PMC8250137/

Maxmen, A., Mallapaty, S. The Covid lab-leak hypothesis: what scientists do and don't know. Nature. June 8, 2021. Accessed January 28, 2023. https://www.nature.com/articles/d41586-021-01529-3

McMahon, D.E., Gallman, A.E., et al. Long Covid in the skin: a registry analysis of Covid-19 dermatological duration. Lancet Infect Dis. 2021 Mar;21(3):313-314. doi: 10.1016/S1473-3099(20)30986-5. Epub 2021 Jan 15. https://pubmed.ncbi.nlm.nih.gov/33460566/

Mehandru, S., Miriam, M. Pathological sequelae of long-haul Covid. Nat Immunol. Author manuscript; available in PMC 2022 May 24. Published in final edited form as: Nat Immunol. 2022 Feb; 23(2): 194–202. Published online 2022 Feb 1. doi: 10.1038/s41590-021-01104-y. https://www.ncbi.nlm.nih.gov/pmc/articles/PMC9127978/

Mu, C., Sheng, Y., et al. Potential compound from herbal food of Rhizoma Polygonati for treatment of Covid-19 analyzed by network pharmacology: Viral and cancer signaling mechanisms. J Funct Foods. 2021 Feb; 77: 104149. Published online 2020 Aug 14. doi: 10.1016/j.jff.2020.104149. https://www.ncbi.nlm.nih.gov/pmc/articles/PMC7427583/

Naughton, S.X., Raval, U., Pasinetti, G.M. Potential Novel Role of Covid-19 in Alzheimer's Disease and Preventative Mitigation Strategies. J Alzheimers Dis. 2020;76(1):21-25. doi: 10.3233/JAD-200537. https://pubmed.ncbi.nlm.nih.gov/32538855/

Oaklander, A.L., Mills, A.J., et al. Peripheral Neuropathy Evaluations of Patients With Prolonged Long Covid. Neurol Neuroimmunol Neuroinflamm. 2022 Mar 1;9(3):e1146. doi: 10.1212/NXI.0000000000001146. Print 2022 May. https://pubmed.ncbi.nlm.nih.gov/35232750/

Ota, K. et al. Effect of Shakuyaku-kanzo-to in patients with muscle cramps: A systematic literature review. J Gen Fam Med. 2020 Feb 16;21(3):56-62. doi: 10.1002/jgf2.302. eCollection 2020 May.

Paidi, R.K., Jana, M., et al. Eugenol, a Component of Holy Basil (Tulsi) and Common Spice Clove, Inhibits the Interaction Between SARS-CoV-2

Spike S1 and ACE2 to Induce Therapeutic Responses. J Neuroimmune Pharmacol. 2021; 16(4): 743–755. Published online 2021 Oct 22. doi: 10.1007/s11481-021-10028-1.
https://www.ncbi.nlm.nih.gov/pmc/articles/PMC8531902/

Parry, P.I., et al.'Spikeopathy': Covid-19 Spike Protein Is Pathogenic, from Both Virus and Vaccine mRNA. Biomedicines. 2023 Aug; 11(8): 2287. Published online 2023 Aug 17. doi: 10.3390/biomedicines11082287

Panda, M., Dash, S., et al. Dermatological Manifestations Associated with Covid-19 Infection. Indian J Dermatol. 2021 May-Jun; 66(3): 237–245. doi: 10.4103/ijd.ijd_464_21.
https://www.ncbi.nlm.nih.gov/pmc/articles/PMC8375538/

Pfizer Responds to Research Claims. Friday, January 27, 2023 - 08:00pm. Accessed January, 29, 2023. https://www.pfizer.com/news/announcements/pfizer-responds-research-claims

Quaglia, M., Merlotti, G., et al. Viral Infections and Systemic Lupus Erythematosus: New Players in an Old Story. Viruses. 2021 Feb; 13(2): 277. Published online 2021 Feb 11. doi: 10.3390/v13020277.
https://www.ncbi.nlm.nih.gov/pmc/articles/PMC7916951/

Rajagopal, K., Varakumar, P., et al. Activity of phytochemical constituents of Curcuma longa (turmeric) and Andrographis paniculata against coronavirus (Covid-19): an in silico approach. Futur J Pharm Sci. 2020; 6(1): 104.Published online 2020 Oct 16. doi: 10.1186/s43094-020-00126-x.
https://www.ncbi.nlm.nih.gov/pmc/articles/PMC7562761/

Rattis, B.A.C., Ramos, S.G., Celes, M.R. Curcumin as a Potential Treatment for Covid-19. Front Pharmacol. 2021; 12: 675287. Published online 2021 May 7. doi: 10.3389/fphar.2021.675287.
https://www.ncbi.nlm.nih.gov/pmc/articles/PMC8138567/

Ren, D., Shen, Z., et al. Pharmacology, phytochemistry, and traditional uses of Scrophularia ningpoensis Hemsl. J Ethnopharmacol. 2021 Apr 6;269:113688. doi: 10.1016/j.jep.2020.113688. Epub 2020 Dec 16.
https://pubmed.ncbi.nlm.nih.gov/33338592/

Sanchez-Ramirez, D.C., Normand, K., et al. Long-Term Impact of Covid-19: A Systematic Review of the Literature and Meta-Analysis. Biomedicines. 2021 Aug; 9(8): 900. Published online 2021 Jul 27. doi: 10.3390/biomedicines9080900.
https://www.ncbi.nlm.nih.gov/pmc/articles/PMC8389585/

Sapkota, H.R., Nune, A. Long Covid from rheumatology perspective — a narrative review. Clin Rheumatol. 2022; 41(2): 337–348. Published online 2021 Nov 30. doi: 10.1007/s10067-021-06001-1. https://www.ncbi.nlm.nih.gov/pmc/articles/PMC8629735/

Sayed, S.E., Gomaa, S., et al. Sleep in post-Covid-19 recovery period and its impact on different domains of quality of life. Egypt J Neurol Psychiatr Neurosurg. 2021;57(1):172. doi: 10.1186/s41983-021-00429-7. Epub 2021 Dec 14. https://pubmed.ncbi.nlm.nih.gov/34924750/

Scheid, V., Bensky D., et al. Chinese Herbal Medicine Formulas and Strategies 2nd Ed. Eastland Press; 2nd edition (March 2, 2009) ISBN-10 : 093961667X

Sehaila, M., Chemat, S. Antimalarial-agent artemisinin and derivatives portray more potent binding to Lys353 and Lys31-binding hotspots of SARS-CoV-2 spike protein than hydroxychloroquine: potential repurposing of artenimol for Covid-19. J Biomol Struct Dyn. 2020 : 1–11.Published online 2020 Jul 22. doi: 10.1080/07391102.2020.1796809. https://www.ncbi.nlm.nih.gov/pmc/articles/PMC7441758/

Shang, Q., Xu, H., et al. Oral Panax notoginseng Preparation for Coronary Heart Disease: A Systematic Review of Randomized Controlled Trials. Evid Based Complement Alternat Med. 2013; 2013: 940125. Published online 2013 Aug 20. doi: 10.1155/2013/940125.. https://www.ncbi.nlm.nih.gov/pmc/articles/PMC3762143/

Shree, P., Mishra, P., et al. Targeting Covid-19 (SARS-CoV-2) main protease through active phytochemicals of ayurvedic medicinal plants – Withania somnifera (Ashwagandha), Tinospora cordifolia (Giloy) and Ocimum sanctum (Tulsi) – a molecular docking study. J Biomol Struct Dyn. 2020 : 1–14. Published online 2020 Aug 27. doi: 10.1080/07391102.2020.1810778. https://www.ncbi.nlm.nih.gov/pmc/articles/PMC7484581/

Song, H., Wang, P., et al. Panax notoginseng Preparations for Unstable Angina Pectoris: A Systematic Review and Meta-Analysis. Phytother Res. 2017 Aug;31(8):1162-1172. doi: 10.1002/ptr.5848. Epub 2017 Jun 20. https://pubmed.ncbi.nlm.nih.gov/28634988/

Stefanou, M., Palaiodimou, L., et al. Neurological manifestations of long-Covid syndrome: a narrative review. Ther Adv Chronic Dis. 2022 Feb 17;13:20406223221076890. doi: 10.1177/20406223221076890. eCollection 2022. https://pubmed.ncbi.nlm.nih.gov/35198136/

Suzuki, Y.J. The viral protein fragment theory of Covid-19 pathogenesis. Med Hypotheses. 2020 Nov; 144: 110267. Published online 2020 Sep 11. doi: 10.1016/j.mehy.2020.110267. https://www.ncbi.nlm.nih.gov/pmc/articles/PMC7485542/

Suzuki, Y.J., Gychna, S.G. SARS-CoV-2 Spike Protein Elicits Cell Signaling in Human Host Cells: Implications for Possible Consequences of Covid-19 Vaccines. Vaccines (Basel). 2021 Jan; 9(1): 36. Published online 2021 Jan 11. doi: 10.3390/vaccines9010036. https://www.ncbi.nlm.nih.gov/pmc/articles/PMC7827936/

Szczuka, D., Nowak, A., et al. American Ginseng (Panax quinquefolium L.) as a Source of Bioactive Phytochemicals with Pro-Health Properties. Nutrients. 2019 May 9;11(5):1041. doi: 10.3390/nu11051041. https://pubmed.ncbi.nlm.nih.gov/31075951/

Tang, W., Tsai, H., et al. Perilla (Perilla frutescens) leaf extract inhibits SARS-CoV-2 via direct virus inactivation. Biomed J. 2021 Jun; 44(3): 293–303. Published online 2021 Jan 28. doi: 10.1016/j.bj.2021.01.005. https://www.ncbi.nlm.nih.gov/pmc/articles/PMC7840404/

Theoharides, T. Could SARS-CoV-2 Spike Protein Be Responsible for Long-Covid Syndrome? Mol Neurobiol. 2022; 59(3): 1850–1861. Published online 2022 Jan 13. doi: 10.1007/s12035-021-02696-0. https://www.ncbi.nlm.nih.gov/pmc/articles/PMC8757925/

Theoharides, T.C., Conti, P. Be aware of SARS-CoV-2 spike protein: There is more than meets the eye. J Biol Regul Homeost Agents. 2021 May-Jun;35(3):833-838. doi: 10.23812/THEO_EDIT_3_21. https://pubmed.ncbi.nlm.nih.gov/34100279/

Theoharides, T., Cholevas, C., et al. Long-Covid syndrome-associated brain fog and chemofog: Luteolin to the rescue. Biofactors. 2021 Mar-Apr; 47(2): 232–241. Published online 2021 Apr 12. doi: 10.1002/biof.1726. https://www.ncbi.nlm.nih.gov/pmc/articles/PMC8250989/

Thimmulappa, R.K., Mudnakudu-Nagaraju, K.K., et al. Antiviral and immunomodulatory activity of curcumin: A case for prophylactic therapy for Covid-19. Heliyon. 2021 Feb; 7(2): e06350. Published online 2021 Feb 22. doi: 10.1016/j.heliyon.2021.e06350. https://www.ncbi.nlm.nih.gov/pmc/articles/PMC7899028/

Tobler, D.L., Pruzansky, A.J., et al. Long-Term Cardiovascular Effects of Covid-19: Emerging Data Relevant to the Cardiovascular Clinician. Curr Atheroscler Rep. 2022 Jul;24(7):563-570. doi: 10.1007/s11883-022-

01032-8. Epub 2022 May 4. https://pubmed.ncbi.nlm.nih.gov/35507278/

Trougakos, I.P., Terpos, E., et al. Adverse effects of Covid-19 mRNA vaccines: the spike hypothesis. Trends Mol Med. 2022 Jul;28(7):542-554. Doi: 10.1016/j.molmed.2022.04.007. Epub 2022 Apr 21. https://pubmed.ncbi.nlm.nih.gov/35537987/

Trougakos, I.P., Terpos, E., et al. Covid-19 mRNA vaccine-induced adverse effects: unwinding the unknowns. Trends Mol Med. 2022 Oct; 28(10): 800–802. Published online 2022 Sep 12. doi: 10.1016/j.molmed.2022.07.008. https://www.ncbi.nlm.nih.gov/pmc/articles/PMC9467519/

Vahedian-Azimi, A., Abbasifard, M., et al. Effectiveness of Curcumin on Outcomes of Hospitalized Covid-19 Patients: A Systematic Review of Clinical Trials. Nutrients. 2022 Jan 7;14(2):256. doi: 10.3390/nu14020256. https://pubmed.ncbi.nlm.nih.gov/35057437/

Van de Sand, L., Bormann, L., et al. Glycyrrhizin Effectively Inhibits SARS-CoV-2 Replication by Inhibiting the Viral Main Protease. Viruses. 2021 Apr; 13(4): 609. Published online 2021 Apr 2. doi: 10.3390/v13040609. https://www.ncbi.nlm.nih.gov/pmc/articles/PMC8066091/

Vanichkachorn, E., Newcomb, R., et al. Persistent circulating SARS-CoV-2 spike is associated with post-acute Covid-19 sequelae. Mayo Clin Proc. 2021 Jul;96(7):1782-1791. doi: 10.1016/j.mayocp.2021.04.024. Epub 2021 May 11. https://pubmed.ncbi.nlm.nih.gov/34218857/

Vicidomini, C., Roviello, V., Roviello, G.N. Molecular Basis of the Therapeutical Potential of Clove (Syzygium aromaticum L.) and Clues to Its Anti-Covid-19 Utility. Molecules. 2021 Apr; 26(7): 1880. Published online 2021 Mar 26. doi: 10.3390/molecules26071880. https://www.ncbi.nlm.nih.gov/pmc/articles/PMC8036487/

Villa, L.L. Viral carcinogenesis: virus implicated in cancer. BMC Proc. 2013; 7(Suppl 2): K11.
Published online 2013 Apr 4. doi: 10.1186/1753-6561-7-S2-K11. https://www.ncbi.nlm.nih.gov/pmc/articles/PMC3624155/

Vlieger, L.D., Vandenbroucke, R.E., Hoecke, L.V. Recent insights into viral infections as a trigger and accelerator in alzheimer's disease. Drug Discov Today. 2022 Aug 18;27(11):103340. doi: 10.1016/j.drudis.2022.103340. https://pubmed.ncbi.nlm.nih.gov/35987492/

Von Borowski, R.G., Trentin, D.S. Biofilms and Coronavirus Reservoirs: a Perspective Review. Appl Environ Microbiol. 2021 Sep; 87(18): e00859-21. Published online 2021 Aug 26. Prepublished online 2021 Jun 30. doi: 10.1128/AEM.00859-21. https://www.ncbi.nlm.nih.gov/pmc/articles/PMC8388801/

Wang, C., Yu, C., et al. Long Covid: The Nature of Thrombotic Sequelae Determines the Necessity of Early Anticoagulation. Front Cell Infect Microbiol. 2022 Apr 5;12:861703. doi: 10.3389/fcimb.2022.861703. eCollection 2022. https://pubmed.ncbi.nlm.nih.gov/35449732/

Wang, J., Wang, L., et al. The isolation, structural features and biological activities of polysaccharide from Ligusticum chuanxiong: A review. Carbohydr Polym. 2022 Jun 1;285:118971. doi: 10.1016/j.carbpol.2021.118971. Epub 2021 Dec 4. https://pubmed.ncbi.nlm.nih.gov/35287839/

Wang, M., Yao, M., et al. Ligusticum chuanxiong exerts neuroprotection by promoting adult neurogenesis and inhibiting inflammation in the hippocampus of ME cerebral ischemia rats. J Ethnopharmacol. 2020 Mar 1;249:112385. doi: 10.1016/j.jep.2019.112385. Epub 2019 Nov 12. https://pubmed.ncbi.nlm.nih.gov/31730888/

Wang, T. Covid-19-Linked Loss of Smell and Taste: Case Study and Discussion. The Journal of Chinese Medicine(Issue 124). October 2020. https://www.journalofchinesemedicine.com/Covid-19-linked-loss-of-smell-and-taste-case-study-and-discussion.html

Wang, X., Lin, S., et al. Polygoni multiflori radix extracts inhibit SARS-CoV-2 pseudovirus entry in HEK293T cells and zebrafish larvae. Phytomedicine. 2022 Jul 20;102:154154. doi: 10.1016/j.phymed.2022.154154. Epub 2022 May 9. https://pubmed.ncbi.nlm.nih.gov/35576740/

Wilcox, L. Translation by Lorraine Wilcox, Gu Toxins. https://www.youtube.com/watch?v=Os9ZZwNh89w

Wouk, J., Rechenchoski, D.Z., et al. Viral infections and their relationship to neurological disorders. Arch Virol. 2021 Mar;166(3):733-753. doi: 10.1007/s00705-021-04959-6. Epub 2021 Jan 27. https://pubmed.ncbi.nlm.nih.gov/33502593/

Wu, Y., et al. Pharmacological effects of Radix Angelica Sinensis (Danggui) on cerebral infarction. Chin Med. 2011; 6: 32. Published online 2011 Aug 25. doi: 10.1186/1749-8546-6-32

Wu, Z., Chen, X., et al. The inhibition of Mpro, the primary protease of Covid-19, by Poria cocos and its active compounds: a network pharmacology and molecular docking study. RSC Adv. 2021 Mar 25;11(20):11821-11843. doi: 10.1039/d0ra07035a. eCollection 2021 Mar 23. https://pubmed.ncbi.nlm.nih.gov/35423770/

Xiao, T., Cui, M., et al. Myricetin Inhibits SARS-CoV-2 Viral Replication by Targeting Mpro and Ameliorates Pulmonary Inflammation. Front Pharmacol. 2021; 12: 669642. Published online 2021 Jun 17. doi: 10.3389/fphar.2021.669642. https://www.ncbi.nlm.nih.gov/pmc/articles/PMC8248548/

Xie, W., Meng, X., et al. Panax Notoginseng Saponins: A Review of Its Mechanisms of Antidepressant or Anxiolytic Effects and Network Analysis on Phytochemistry and Pharmacology. Molecules. 2018 Apr 17;23(4):940. doi: 10.3390/molecules23040940. https://pubmed.ncbi.nlm.nih.gov/29673237/

Xu, Y., Tan, H., et al. Panax notoginseng for Inflammation-Related Chronic Diseases: A Review on the Modulations of Multiple Pathways. Am J Chin Med. 2018;46(5):971-996. doi: 10.1142/S0192415X18500519. Epub 2018 Jul 5. https://pubmed.ncbi.nlm.nih.gov/29976083/

Yang, F., Ma, Q., et al. Panax notoginseng for Cerebral Ischemia: A Systematic Review. Am J Chin Med. 2020;48(6):1331-1351. doi: 10.1142/S0192415X20500652. Epub 2020 Sep 9. https://pubmed.ncbi.nlm.nih.gov/32907361/

Yang, L., Hou, A., et al. Panacis Quinquefolii Radix: A Review of the Botany, Phytochemistry, Quality Control, Pharmacology, Toxicology and Industrial Applications Research Progress. Front Pharmacol. 2020; 11: 602092. Published online 2020 Dec 8. doi: 10.3389/fphar.2020.602092. https://www.ncbi.nlm.nih.gov/pmc/articles/PMC7768635/

Yang, M., Xue, L., et al. Ethnopharmacology, Phytochemistry, and Pharmacology of the Genus Glehnia: A Systematic Review. Evid Based Complement Alternat Med. 2019; 2019: 1253493. Published online 2019 Dec 14. doi: 10.1155/2019/1253493. https://www.ncbi.nlm.nih.gov/pmc/articles/PMC6931029/

Yeh, Y., Doan, L.H., et al. Honeysuckle (Lonicera japonica) and Huangqi (Astragalus membranaceus) Suppress SARS-CoV-2 Entry and Covid-19 Related Cytokine Storm in Vitro. Front Pharmacol. 2022 Mar

25;12:765553. doi: 10.3389/fphar.2021.765553. eCollection 2021. https://pubmed.ncbi.nlm.nih.gov/35401158/

Yonker, L.M., Swank, Z., et al. Circulating Spike Protein Detected in Post-Covid-19 mRNA Vaccine Myocarditis. Circulation. 2023 Jan 4. Doi: 10.1161/CIRCULATIONAHA.122.061025. Online ahead of print. https://pubmed.ncbi.nlm.nih.gov/36597886/

Zhao, H., Feng, Y., et al. Bai Zhi (Angelica Dahuricae Radix). Front Pharmacol. 2022 Jul 1;13:896637. doi: 10.3389/fphar.2022.896637. eCollection 2022. https://pubmed.ncbi.nlm.nih.gov/35847034/

Zhao, H., Zeng, S., et al. Lonicerae Japonicae Flos Attenuates Neutrophilic Inflammation by Inhibiting Oxidative Stress. Curr Opin Pharmacol. 2021 Oct;60:200-207. doi: 10.1016/j.coph.2021.07.019. Epub 2021 Aug 10. https://pubmed.ncbi.nlm.nih.gov/36139855/

Zhao, H., Zeng, S., et al. Updated pharmacological effects of Lonicerae japonicae flos, with a focus on its potential efficacy on coronavirus disease-2019 (Covid-19). Curr Opin Pharmacol. 2021 Oct;60:200-207. doi: 10.1016/j.coph.2021.07.019. Epub 2021 Aug 10. https://pubmed.ncbi.nlm.nih.gov/34461565/

Zhang, H., Huang., L., et al. An Overview of Systematic Reviews of Ginkgo biloba Extracts for Mild Cognitive Impairment and Dementia. Front Aging Neurosci. 2016; 8: 276. Published online 2016 Dec 6. doi: 10.3389/fnagi.2016.00276. https://www.ncbi.nlm.nih.gov/pmc/articles/PMC5138224/

Zhang, Q., Huang, H., et al. Traditional Uses, Pharmacological Effects, and Molecular Mechanisms of Licorice in Potential Therapy of Covid-19. Front Pharmacol. 2021 Nov 26;12:719758. doi: 10.3389/fphar.2021.719758. eCollection 2021. https://pubmed.ncbi.nlm.nih.gov/34899289/

Zhang, Q., Liu, A., Wang, Y. Scrophularia ningpoensis Hemsl: a review of its phytochemistry, pharmacology, quality control and pharmacokinetics. J Pharm Pharmacol. 2021 Mar 27;73(5):573-600. doi: 10.1093/jpp/rgaa036. https://pubmed.ncbi.nlm.nih.gov/33772290/

Zharkikh, E.V., et al. Assessment of Blood Microcirculation Changes after Covid-19 Using Wearable Laser Doppler Flowmetry. Diagnostics (Basel). 2023 Mar; 13(5): 920. Published online 2023 Mar 1. doi: 10.3390/diagnostics13050920

Zheng, Q., Zhuang, Z., et al. Clinical and Preclinical Systematic Review of Astragalus Membranaceus for Viral Myocarditis. Oxid Med Cell

Longev. 2020 Nov 2;2020:1560353. doi: 10.1155/2020/1560353. eCollection 2020. https://pubmed.ncbi.nlm.nih.gov/33204391/

Zhong, H., Xue, X., et al. Integrated analysis of the chemical-material basis and molecular mechanisms for the classic herbal formula of Lily Bulb and Rehmannia Decoction in alleviating depression. Chin Med. 2021 Oct 21;16(1):107. doi: 10.1186/s13020-021-00519-x. https://pubmed.ncbi.nlm.nih.gov/34674715/

www.ingramcontent.com/pod-product-compliance
Lightning Source LLC
Chambersburg PA
CBHW071121160426
43196CB00013B/2659